Advance Praise for

What's Your Diet Type?

"Eating well and living healthily—though vital—does not have a one-size-fits-all prescription. Heather K. Jones, by using Diet Types, now empowers each of us—using our own language and learning strategies—to get healthy. The marriage of personality type and diet is long overdue!"

—Hile Rutledge, CEO, OKA (Otto Kroeger Associates)

"No more one-size-fits-all diets! This book gives every dieter what she really needs: A personalized plan for weight loss—and the tools, tips and recipes that will help her reach her goal."

—Pam O'Brien, Executive Editor, *Fitness* magazine

"Heather K. Jones' upbeat and practical diet guide taps into the key to diet success: finding a plan that fits you and your life! Readers will see themselves in the Types Jones describes, discover their weight loss strengths and find doable solutions to their specific diet trip-ups. We all know what to do to lose those pounds, Jones tells you how."

— Erin Hobday, Diet & Nutrition Editor at *SELF* Magazine

"This eye-opening book will help you understand yourself and your eating habits a lot better. And that's key when looking to find a long-term diet strategy that works for you!"

— Lisa "Hungry Girl" Lillien

DISCLAIMER

The Diet Type program is not designed to, and does not provide, medical advice. This book and its program are intended as a reference and informational volume only, not as a medical manual. The Diet Type program is not intended as a substitute for the advice and/or medical care of your physician, nor is it meant to discourage or dissuade you from the advice of your physician. You should regularly consult with a physician in matters relating to your health, especially with regard to symptoms that may require diagnosis. Any lifestyle change should be undertaken under the direct supervision of your physician.

If you have any questions concerning the information presented in this program, or its application to your medical profile, or if you have any medical, nutritional, or psychological needs or constraints that may conflict with the information in this program, you should consult with your physician before beginning the program. The Diet Type program contains only the author(s) opinions, thoughts and conclusions. Again, it is for educational purposes only, and you, and only you, are responsible if you choose to do anything based on what you read, hear, or see. Should you choose to make use of the information contained herein without first consulting a health professional, you are prescribing for yourself, which is your right; however, the author(s) and publisher(s) do not assume any responsibility whatsoever under any conditions or circumstances for your actions and choices.

Your use of this program creates a legal and binding agreement that you will hold us harmless for any decisions you make or harm that may come to yourself or others, directly or indirectly. The Diet Type program is purely informational, and how you choose to use this information is solely at your own risk. The Diet Type program assumes no liability for anything that happens as a result of your use of this program. In no event shall the Diet Type program or their affiliates, employees, agents, content providers, or licensors be liable for any indirect, consequential, special, incidental, or punitive damages related to the content or any errors or omissions in the content.

The case studies, quotes, and biographical facts presented are actual and true-to-life, they are compilations of the thousands of patient interactions, survey results, and direct interviews performed by the authors. The names of all individuals mentioned in the case studies have been altered to protect privacy.

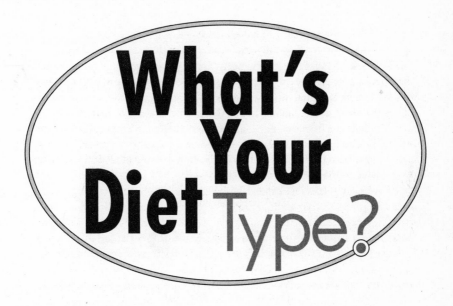

What's Your Diet Type?

HEATHER K. JONES, R.D.

WITH MARY MISCISIN, M.S. AND ED REDARD, M.D.

hatherleigh

PEA Member   Recycled Content   Earth-Friendly Printing

5-22 46th Avenue, Suite 200
Long Island City, NY 11101
www.hatherleighpress.com

Library of Congress Cataloging-in-Publication Data

Jones, Heather K.
 What's your diet type? / by Heather K. Jones, with Mary Miscisin, and Ed
Redard.
  p. cm.
 ISBN 978-1-57826-287-8 (alk. paper)
 1. Weight loss—Psychological aspects. 2. Personality. I. Miscisin, Mary. II.
Redard, Ed. III. Title.
 RM222.2.J617 2008
 613.2'5—dc22
         2008040084

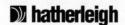

To my Planner, Aaron.
Without your love and support this book
would not have been possible.
—HEATHER

Contents

Acknowledgements

S PECIAL THANKS TO Aaron Haesler, Tamara Goldis, R.D.; Beth Sumrell Ehrensberger, M.P.H., R.D.; Jennifer Curtis; June Eding; Anna Krusinski; Ryan Tumambing; Mary Woodward; Danielle Hazard; Namita Davis; Deborah Cohen, M.H.Sc., R.D.; Lauren Clark, R.D.; Andrea Au Levitt; Janis Jibrin, M.S., R.D.; Tracy Olgeaty Gensler M.S., R.D.; Jean Marie Miscisin; Crescentia Miscisin; Therese Schaaf; Tamela Moore; Lori Brennan; Cyndi McClave; Mary Jones; Janice Whiting; Louise Kutz; Diane Blair; Tim Hallbom; Kris Hallbom; Michelle Fong; Marie Elizabeth; Paulette Briggs; Victoria Laluz; Manuel Gill; Dave Eshe; Lisa Powers; Christine Troyano; Anthony Robbins; Richard Bandler; Don Lowry; Erica Lowry; and Mercy Medical Foundation.

A special appreciation goes to Otto Kroeger for his pioneering efforts and expertise in the ever expanding field of typology and for writing the foreword to this book; to Hile Rutledge, CEO of Otto Kroeger Associates; to all of the thousands of people who participated in the weight management survey and the participants of Mary's "A Colorful Approach to Weight Management" workshops, who contributed their opinions, preferences and personality approaches; to many of Dr. Redard's patients, whose names cannot be mentioned out of confidentiality; and to my agent Janis Donnaud, for believing in this book.

Foreword
– Otto Kroeger –

F YOU'VE EVER been discouraged about keeping your weight in control... if you've ever thought dieting successfully is a hopeless cause... if you've ever been over fed with the wrong food... if you are "fed up" with diet programs... if you are convinced that diets are intentionally made to be complicated and difficult just so you'll grow weary and fail... then this book is for you. *What's Your Diet Type?* confronts, simplifies, and overcomes all these issues, and will give you the hope and encouragement you need to change your eating habits, drop pounds, and live healthfully. How? By helping you find a diet made just for your personality—yes: *custom-made* for your own unique personality.

As an expert on the Myers-Briggs Type Indicator® (MBTI®) and co-author of four leading books on Type: *Type Talk, Type Talk At Work, 16 Ways to Love Your Lover,* and *Personality Type and Religious Leadership,* I have travelled the world sharing my knowledge on personality and guiding people to an understanding of the way personality shapes everything they do. At presentations for personal and professional groups, I have enabled participants to tap into their own strengths and navigate their weaknesses, so they could achieve maximum success, no matter what their goal.

The power of personality applies to the goal of weight loss, too. Our personality is so integrated with *how* and *what* we eat that failure to engage our personality preferences when we try to control our weight sets us up for weight *gain* rather than weight *loss*. It is like someone who is right-handed being forced to use their left hand; the result is frustration and wasted effort.

This book in a refreshing and affirming way changes all that. In the first part of the book, a detailed overview of personality differences helps us understand what our own personal nuances are all about, and how they shape our lives. Then, Heather explains how you can create a tailormade eating and dieting plan that will work with your personal strengths and carefully work around your weaknesses. As you look closer at your strengths, and build upon them, you will come to an even more powerful understanding of how your natural physical and psychological motivations influence your efforts at weight control. You will be reminded that strategies that may have helped a friend or mate may even work *against* you, because they work against your own personal attributes. Though based on a rather complex personality system, Heather's free-flowing style is easy to follow, and she presents a variety of different dieting styles for each personality type. With encouragement and sensitivity, she is accepting of slip-ups, and, at the same time, presents strategies to help you get back on the path to success. Heather compliments her close study of personality types with inspired eating strategies and work out plans. With your efforts to link *who you are* to *how you live*—and that includes what you do and what you eat—and Heather's inspired tips and plans, you will attain your goal.

This book is just the partner you need on your journey towards good eating and healthy living habits—habits that work in sync with the unique individual that you are. You are what you eat, but you hold the power to decide *how* you eat, too.

OTTO KROEGER
Fairfax, VA, 2008

Introductions

Heather's Story: A Diet Player

Before we take a closer look at who *you* are, what your goals are, and how we will make reaching those goals a part of your life, I'll tell you a little about myself.

I am a registered dietitian, health advocate, weight loss counselor, nutrition writer, and freelance health journalist who has spent the last decade assisting people who struggle with weight management and food issues. I have spent seven of those years working for the *Nutrition Action Healthletter,* the nation's largest circulation health newsletter. I'm also a nutrition consultant for *The Best Life Diet* by Bob Greene, who is Oprah's personal fitness trainer. I am passionate about my health, and I make sure to get lots of exercise, eat my fruits and vegetables, get plenty of whole grains, and drink lots of water.

But...

I am also a foodie! A foodie is defined as "a person who has an ardent or refined interest in food." Well, that's me! I love food and I love to eat food. In fact, in high school I was voted "the girl with the biggest appetite." That's right. No run of the mill "most likely to succeed" or "best smile" class superlative for me. Instead, I was designated as the person who really, really likes food. And I do! Specifically, bacon. I LOVE bacon! Oh, and I don't want to forget pasta and cheese. Did I mention chocolate and crème brulee? The list goes on and on, and I am sure I will add more to it before the year is over—I love food so much that I travel the globe just to try more of it. Spanish tapas, French pastries, and Thai curries, just to name a few... YUM! I also love trying new restaurants, and I've been known to spend hours in specialty food stores, carefully selecting rich imported cheeses and fine chocolates to try. I even spent a year working for a gourmet catering company, planning parties and menus that featured incredibly fabulous and totally decadent dishes. I subscribe to *Bon Appétit*, *Gourmet*, and *Cooking Light*, and I love the Bravo TV show "Top Chef."

So just how does a registered dietitian and a self-proclaimed "foodie" manage to combine her passion for health and food and stay healthy and fit?

This is a good question—and one that I am asked ALL the time! In fact, it is the "answer" to that question that inspired me to write this book.

The Answer

When women find out I work in the weight loss biz, the first question out of their mouths is usually, "so what's the secret to losing weight, and keeping it off?" They're convinced I hold the key to the kingdom of skinny-dom, and they want to know what I do, how I do it, how I can help them—fast!

But the truth is, these women shouldn't be asking me about me. Instead, they should be asking themselves about who they are. That's because what works for me may not necessarily work for them. Simply put: one size does not fit all in the world of weight loss. Dieting and healthy living is not a mathematical problem with one single solution. Why? Because healthy exercise and eating habits can only be attained by the person who is striving for them, and whoever that person is, he or she is totally unique. That means they need a dieting and eating approach that is as unique and special as they are.

Think about it: we all have different personalities, with specific preferences and priorities, thoughts and feelings, and ways of doing things. It only makes sense that we would require our own, one-of-a-kind, eating, exercising, and dieting plan, too.

For example, while a free-flowing, flexible diet approach that provides lifestyle solutions for people who live "in the moment" works best for my personality (I'm a Diet Player), some would find this loosey-goosey plan completely frustrating and unworkable. Trying to lose weight in a way that doesn't match your personality is like trying to squeeze yourself into a pair of shoes that are two sizes too small: it takes more work than it should, it's very uncomfortable, and you won't be able to get anywhere!

So how do you find the healthy weight loss methods that work for you? By working with your personality!

What My Mother Taught Me

The idea that we don't all come from the same cookie cutter is something I was introduced to at an early age. In addition to making sure me and my two sisters ate well (fresh fruits instead of frosted cereal, crisp veggies instead of chips, and no soda) my "supermom" also encouraged us to be healthy on the inside by exploring our innermost selves. When my sisters and I were teenagers, my mom came across the Myers-Briggs Type Indicator (MBTI®) in one of her many self-help psychology books. For my mom, this was the perfect tool to help guide her daughters towards becoming (in her words) "authentic individuals." So she promptly got us to take the quiz. But we didn't notice that we were on a journey of self-discovery—we were too busy having fun!

The MBTI® assessment was thrilling and exciting to us because so much about our personalities was right there in the book. It was almost like having a mind reader! My sisters, my mom and I would sit around for hours, gleefully describing our quirks to each other and discussing our personality types.

But the MBTI® was, and is, more than just fun and games. Personality typing is a powerful and respected method of identifying and understanding a person's true and inherent nature. It is based on more than sixty years of scientific research, and it is the most widely used personality examination in the world.

So when I decided to take a closer look at the key to effective weight loss, I automatically turned to what I knew about personality.

The MBTI® Connection

When I began combining my knowledge of nutrition with the concepts of personality typing (I'm a certified MBTI® administrator) and customizing my diet advice, the results were astounding! I learned that certain eating and exercise strategies worked so well for others they were almost effortless—while others failed completely. I knew that these vast differences meant I had hit on something powerful.

Soon, I reached out to two of my favorite personality experts, Mary Miscisin and Ed Redard, for their take on the personality/dieting connection. As it turns out, I couldn't have picked more perfect contributors.

Mary Miscisin, the author of *Showing Our True Colors*, is a personality specialist who regularly presents at national conferences. During her presentations, Mary had been grouping her workshop participants according to four personality styles and then having them design their ideal weight management course. With the expertise of Ed Redard, a family practice physician, they were already exploring the personality and weight loss link.

The Research

Participants eagerly responded to Mary's interactive presentations on personality patterns and weight loss, and Mary and Dr. Redard developed a system so that they could repeat personality/weight loss strategies in session after session. As they further customized each participant's plan to their personality, the positive results increased even more.

After seeing such incredible results with the workshop participants, Dr. Redard began using the concepts in his practice to help patients with weight management challenges. First, he designed a survey that helped him identify the patient's personality type and history of diet habits. Then, he used this information to customize "diet prescriptions." Once again, the results were amazing. Patients for whom nothing had ever worked were suddenly making huge progress.

Together, we decided to take it even further. Focus groups were held at local bookstores to test the validity of Dr. Redard's "diet prescriptions." Professionals and colleagues were interviewed, an on-line version of the original survey was designed, and over 6,000 responses were received. The result? Our research confirmed that each personality style had very different approaches to managing their weight, and that knowing this is the key to finding the best way to lose weight, eat healthy, and feel great. There is no way around it—you have to work with yourself if you are going to win the weight loss battle!

Type and temperament experts such as Otto Kroeger had already been gathering data about different personalities' approaches to weight management, and fitness and nutrition professionals (like myself) had been matching up clients' personalities with exercise and dieting recommendations for years. Yet, out of the hundreds of diet books on my shelves, not one made this important connection. Mary, Dr. Redard, and I realized we would be the first to write a book on this important topic.

The book you are holding in your hands right now is backed up by actual case studies, and features quotes and stories from real patients (the names of all individuals have been altered to protect privacy). The facts and personality insights are compilations of the thousands of survey results and one-on-one interviews. This book is an ideal tool for you to use to unlock the power of your personality, and achieve your weight loss and healthy living goals—for life.

So what are you waiting for? Let's get started on making this book work for you! How? All you need to do is answer one simple question.

The Question

What is the question that holds the key to success? It's so important that it is the title of this book... it is:

What's Your Diet Type?

Are you an organized and responsible Diet Planner, an adventurous and adaptable Diet Player, a passionate and idealistic Diet Feeler, or an intellectual and independent Diet Thinker? Just take the simple quiz inside, based on the MBTI®, and you'll find your answer. Then, you can tap into the power of your personality to achieve the weight goals you desire and deserve, help you fight disease, increase energy, and feel great!

The insightful personality profiles, customized weight loss advice and plans, lifestyle guidance, and real case studies will guide you to success. You'll learn what every Diet Type needs to know about the basics of food, nutrition, and weight loss, enabling you to make wiser daily food, nutrition, and fitness decisions.

No matter who you are, this book is what you've been waiting for! Whether you're a new mom struggling to take off the baby weight or a busy career gal looking for quick solutions, whether this is your first try at weight control or your 100th, whether you want to lose 5 pounds, or 50, whether your goal is weight loss or weight maintenance... this book will equip you with the powerful insight and necessary answers you need to lose weight, get healthy and feel good—forever.

What's Your Diet Type? is not about going "on" a restricted diet, cutting out the foods you love, or depriving yourself. It's about implementing healthy solutions and making comfortable changes that fit easily into your life, and that will work *for* life.

What's Your Diet Type? will...

- Show you how your personality affects the way you eat, exercise, and approach weight loss so you can take back control.
- Teach you the habits, mindset, and challenges of your personality so you can overcome them with workable and sustainable lifestyle solutions.
- Show you how to take advantage of your unique strengths so you can reduce stress, feel better, and truly enjoy a healthier way of living.
- Help you develop your personal, one-of-a-kind lifetime plan so you can look your best—and finally get back into your "skinny" jeans!

Mary's Story: A Diet Feeler
...in her own words

Like a lot of women, my weight did not become an issue until I became a mother. However, it wasn't losing weight right after my daughter was born that tripped me up (I got lucky and lost that relatively quickly). In fact, it wasn't until my daughter was five years old that the "baby weight" caught up with me...literally! I stepped on the scale and realized that the number matched my weight when I was nine months pregnant. My weight had slowly been increasing over the years, but it wasn't until that moment that it hit me. For the first time, I looked in the mirror and really saw how much weight I had gained.

It was the Eighties at the time, and "low fat" was the diet of the moment. So I cut all fats from my diet: no cheese on pizza, no sour cream on baked potato, no butter on toast. As the fat on and in my food decreased, my appetite increased. So I turned to delicious, fat-free baked goods. I thought, "as long as there's no fat, it's healthy!" as I polished off a cinnamon swirl pastry and an apple strudel. I was an avid label reader who only looked at one thing: the fat content. In my mind, less fat meant healthier.

But all that label-reading and careful adherence to the fat-free was to no avail. In fact, I gained five more pounds! On top of that, I was constantly ravenous and drained of energy (of course there was only way to replenish that energy—more sugar). As the numbers on the scale got higher and higher, I started getting migraines. I felt completely out of control, and the situation took its toll on my emotions as I berated myself almost constantly about how awful I looked.

I finally admitted that I had to get help. So I decided to consult a hypnotist. I wanted him to make me hate sugar! But he refused to hypnotize me until I saw a doctor. And it's a good thing he did. The check-up revealed that my blood sugar was so low that I should have been in a coma! It turns out I had created a vicious cycle of consuming high quantities of sugar, getting an insulin rush that, once it crashed, pushed my blood sugar even lower and made me crave even more sugar. My doctor put me on a diet of six small, high protein means a day—with fat! He explained that the fat slows the absorption of sugar into my blood stream, and that it was a necessity in order for my body to function properly.

Almost immediately after changing my diet per my doctor's advice, my headaches dissipated and my energy returned. I felt so rejuvenated! And soon enough, I started losing weight—the healthy way.

Fascinated by the drama I had endured, I decided to pursue a Bachelor's degree in Fitness. Because my emotions had been so intertwined with my weight loss struggles, I also decided to obtain a Master's in Behavior Change. After graduation, I began teaching weight management classes. I noticed that, often, a behavior modification technique that would work for one person, would fail for another. Why, I wondered? The question continued to haunt me during my work as a Wellness Program Coordinator and University health instructor.

Then, one day, I attended a National Wellness Conference and was introduced to the concepts of temperament and personality through a session called True Colors©. I was hooked! Soon, I became certified to teach the True Colors© program so that I could share it with everyone. At the same time, I continued researching temperament and became a qualified Myers Briggs Type Indicator® administrator. With this new knowledge, I finally felt that I understood how a personality type can affect weight management and weight loss. This was why a method that is effective for one person, doesn't work for another! I incorporated what I had learned into my own life as well as into my classes, and, over time, I successfully "followed" my personality type (I'm a Diet Feeler) to a healthy lifestyle and a healthy weight.

In 2001, my book, *Showing Our True Colors*, was published. By this time, my associate, Ed Redard, was also certified to teach True Colors©. He integrated the concepts into his medical practice to help patients unlock their own personal motivation to lose weight. Together, we researched and collected information about True Colors© and its important role in weight loss.

One day, we received a call from Heather, who informed us that she wanted to write a book about temperaments and successful weight loss, and that she would like to feature our research and utilize our expertise to make the project as successful as possible. It was obvious that combining our talents would lead to a powerful and effective book and that sharing our knowledge would be incredibly rewarding. So we joined Heather in creating *What's Your Diet Type?* Now, it's up to you finish the story!

For *you* are the most important part of this book. You will bring your own unique circumstances and personality traits with you on this journey. Along the way you will deepen your understanding of healthy eating habits, and come to know yourself better than you ever thought possible. Finally, you will be able to take what you have learned to achieve, and maintain, your ultimate goals—whether it is losing weight, eating well, living healthy, or looking and feeling great.

Before you begin your journey, think about what you want to accomplish.

Got it?

Now, prepare yourself for the adventure of a lifetime!

Dr. Redard's Story: A Diet Thinker
...in his own words

As a practicing physician, people have come to me with countless questions. Still, there are two questions that come up again and again—"how do I lose weight?" and "how can I keep it off?" If you think about it, the question could also translate to "how do I change for the better, and how can I stick with it?" People are often surprised to know that I too, have been haunted by these questions.

At a young age I had the distinct awareness that I was "different" than the rest of the kids at school. I found playing with others stressful, and found more joy looking at blades of grass through a microscope, or studying the clouds and weather patterns. Looking back, I can see that I was simply a "geek" in training, but back then it was confusing, uncomfortable, and even outright depressing to believe I was so different. Although my teachers praised me for my intellectual accomplishments, it was a shallow reward. I would have given anything to be like one of the cool kids, to fit in. Nowadays I would have probably been labeled as clinically depressed, but at that time all I can recall is feeling a profound emptiness.

Around the 5th grade I began to fill this void with food. Eating would almost miraculously take me into momentary bliss, melting away my troubles and filling the emptiness. The only problem was that food only filled this "emptiness" temporarily. Using my scientific mind I generated a unique solution to this dilemma. Eat more, and eat more often—and to a certain point this strategy actually worked. The only problem was that this strategy had some unexpected consequences. By the sixth grade I weighed 200 pounds, and by the seventh grade I weighed over 250 pounds, wore size 44 pants, and had picked up the habit of hiding food (in my locker, under my bed, around the house). Although I intellectually understood that eating wasn't giving me what I really wanted, it was a method to happiness I felt competent in performing.

Food would have been a perfect solution if it weren't for those nagging side effects: stretch marks, tiredness, and being scorned, put down, and made fun of by all of those "judgmental people." It has been said that change happens when where you are is more painful than where you need to be, and so it was true for me. In a moment of clarity I understood that there must be an answer, there must be a solution, and there must be a method to lose weight and "fit in."

So off to the library I went to read and research all the current diet books. I immediately began to implement their suggestions and exercise plans, while keeping a chart of my progress. It was actually easier than I had thought—in 4 months I lost 40 lbs and by the end of the year I had lost 60 lbs.

Entering college proved to be another difficult time in my life. Although my weight was now down to 185 pounds, I was still feeling that nagging sense that I didn't fit in, that I was different. I thought, "wow, I must still be overweight!" Since dieting and exercise had worked so well in the past, simply doing more of it should help pull me out of my slump, right? Well, it seemed logical at the time. I instituted my plan by upping my running mileage, skipping breakfast and lunch and only eating a salad for dinner. My weight plummeted, leveling out at 160 pounds. I was tired, couldn't concentrate, and had frequent headaches, but at least I was thinner...and thinner meant I would fit in, people would like me, and I would feel normal. But it backfired. My roommates were constantly asking if I was alright, my parents feared I had contracted a serious disease, and my brother joked that I was going for the "hostage look." One day I had pictures taken for my medical school application and when I first saw them, I was horrified. I had seen myself in recent pictures, but I hadn't really *seen* myself. In these pictures I did indeed look emaciated, I *did* look sick. In a reflective moment, I realized that how and what I ate wasn't the answer, and neither was how much exercise I did...there just had to be another solution to this dilemma and I was going to find it!

I headed back to the book store, although this time I didn't go to the diet section, I went to the self-help section instead. I picked up *Your Erroneous Zones* by Wayne Dyer, *A Guide to Rational Living* by Albert Ellis, and many others. I found many of their ideas useful and accurate, but it wasn't until my first year of medical school that I received the self-help I really needed. That year we took the MBTI®, and it turned out to be the answer I was looking for. The MBTI® revealed that I was an INTP, which translates into a Diet Thinker. As I read the lengthy description of my type, it was as though I was reading my own diary! It was like someone had been following me around for the last 20 years, describing what was going on in my head! I am not exactly sure why, but at that moment my search for "self" ended. I finally realized that all of my idiosyncrasies did not make me abnormal or deficient, it was just who I was.

Now I am not sure that you'll have the same sort of life-changing experience when you discover your specific Diet Type. But one thing is certain—you are not alone. Whatever your diet history has been, whatever successes or failures you may have had, there are other people in this world that have had similar experiences. More importantly, there are others that have had similar experiences and still achieved the results they wanted. For me, this was the additional power of Diet Types—that I wouldn't have to struggle through this alone, and that I can benefit from the wisdom of those that have gone before me—and so it is for you too. With the tools and insights I had learned from personality typing, maintaining my ideal weight became less of a struggle and instead felt more like a "project" I managed on a daily basis. Instead of weight control feeling like struggling to catch the last gasp of air on a sinking ship, it became more like balancing a checkbook—making sure that everything was in order and balanced at the end of the day. Sure, at first that checkbook just had to be balanced by bedtime; but as time went on it was okay if I was a few cents over or a few cents under because, over time, things became "reconciled."

My natural curiosity propelled me on a journey to discover even more tools that could facilitate change, even in "resistant" people. I became a Master Practitioner of Neuro-Linguistic Programming, Ericksonian Hypnosis, a certified True Colors© Trainer, and a certified MBTI® administrator. Through using these tools for the past 20 years in medical practice and by observing thousands struggle, gain control, and then obtain their weight goals, I can tell you a few things for certain: that you are not wrong, broken or even unique in your circumstance; that, inherent in your personality, you already have all the resources you need to achieve the results you desire; that you may have "failed" in the past does not make you a failure, but has only given you valuable information to help make your next effort more likely to succeed; that achieving your weight goal is not the end, but the beginning of a whole new adventure in your life.

The hope and goal of this program is that you not only achieve the weight you want, desire, and deserve, but also that you use the tools you are about to learn to become an even more happy, giving, and productive person of this world—and have fun doing it! I have the utmost respect for you for joining us on this journey. I know from personal experience that your determination, courage and tenacity will be well rewarded. I hope our paths cross soon so you can share your success!

PART ONE

Your Personality

CHAPTER 1
Personality and Health

The Skinny

Have you ever wondered why some women have no trouble being healthy and maintaining an ideal weight, while others run in circles, going from one new diet, exercise gimmick, or weight loss fad to another? Do some women have more motivation, willpower, or determination than others? Have some uncovered the mysterious metabolic secret for staying thin and trim? Or can some lucky ladies eat and drink whatever they want, without ever gaining a pound?

What "secret" do the successful women have that the others don't?

Here's your answer: the women who succeed have simply discovered which weight loss approaches and healthy lifestyle solutions work for them and their own unique personalities.

Our personality affects all facets of our lives—from the subjects that we like in school, to how we act in social settings, to the professions and careers we find fulfilling. It also determines why some diet and health approaches work for us, while others fail. While one person enjoys counting calories or points, another cringes at the idea. Whereas some like the flexibility of food choices, others overeat when they're faced with too many decisions. That's why a weight loss approach that's helpful for your sister, neighbor, best friend, or coworker won't necessarily work for you. It's not your metabolism, your genetics, or your love of pasta that's getting you off track and keeping you from losing weight. You simply *can't* succeed at a weight loss approach if your own unique personality does not "sync up" with that particular diet. And while you can't change your personality, you *can* change your strategy!

So, *how* do you find the right approach for you? *Find your Diet Type.*

THE *RIGHT* WAY

Years of research and observation by myself and my co-authors have shown that overcoming the diet/dieter mismatch is key. When the "right" approach is matched with the "right" person, success is a sure thing. The right approach will end years of yo-yo dieting and weight loss struggles. The right approach will work with your schedule and compliment the way you live. The right approach will take advantage of your strengths and help you build healthy habits that will fit effortlessly into your lifestyle. The right approach will work *for* you because it will be personally fulfilling *to* you. Simply put: *the right approach will work.*

What's a Diet Type?

Diet Types are based on methods of classifying personalities found in the Myers-Briggs Type Indicator® (MBTI®), an effective tool for uncovering personality that has been used in workplaces and classrooms around the world for over 60 years. Just as each one of us is either right or left-handed, everyone has an inborn personality type, and although our capability to change and evolve physically, emotionally, mentally, and spiritually is limitless, our inborn personality type does not change significantly over a lifetime.

All "Diets" are Not Created Equal

So do different personalities need different foods? Do some Diet Types need to eat more whole grains while others should avoid, say, beans and citrus fruits? Or should one Diet Type fill up on protein, while for another it's carbohydrates?

Absolutely not!

While many weight loss plans want you to believe that eating specific foods or combinations of nutrients will help you lose weight faster and burn fat more efficiently, or that different foods work better for different people depending on their physiological make-up, the truth is that a good weight loss plan will teach you sound nutrition basics and how to incorporate them into your lifestyle. You need to seek out an approach that is not only healthy, but also a good fit for you personally.

How to Read This Book

People will read this book in different ways. Some might read it from the first page to the last, while others will turn directly to their own Diet Type chapter and ignore the rest. And still others will just skip around and read at their pleasure—after all, this book is packed full of good stuff! Ultimately, your choice depends largely on (yup, you got it!) your personality. It's a good idea to read this book whatever way you feel most comfortable, however, one thing is an absolute "must" if you want to get the most out of the important tool you hold in your hands.

No matter what your Diet Type, *you must read The Basics in Chapter 7.* The endless supply of contradictory diet and health books on the market today, the influx of confusing nutrition advice—along with the plethora of diet pills, patches, gimmicks, and fads—make it nearly impossible for people to separate weight loss fact from fiction. The Basics are a trustworthy

SIFTING THROUGH THE SCIENCE

The type system originated from the work of Carl Jung and was later expanded upon and refined by Katherine Briggs and her daughter, Isabel Myers. Jung, a Swiss psychoanalyst, was among the first academics to view an individual in terms of their patterns of behavior. Myers and Briggs adapted Jung's theory and devised the Myers-Briggs Type Indicator (MBTI®). Later, psychologist David Keirsey distilled the work of Myers and Briggs by grouping the sixteen MBTI® personality *types* into four main personality *temperaments.* An educator named Don Lowry studied under Keirsey and immediately saw the potential for temperament theory to be applied in schools and businesses towards maximizing productivity, and to be used by everyday individuals to help them gain a deeper understanding of themselves. Lowry assigned a color to each temperament, simplified much of the complicated psychological language, and reorganized it all into a system called True Colors©. Because True Colors© is easy to learn and remember, and the results can be used immediately, it quickly became popular.

For more on the True Colors© methodology, I would highly recommend the foundational book *Showing Our True Colors©* by my co-author, Mary Miscisin, a recognized authority on True Colors©.

TEMPERAMENTS THROUGH THE TIMES

The temperament theory is not new. Modern and ancient philosophers as well as psychologists have grouped people into four temperaments. Take a look:

Hippocrates	Melancholic	Sanguine	Phlegmatic	Choleric
Aristotle	Propietary	Hedonic	Ethical	Dialectical
Keirsey	Guardians (SJ)	Artisans (SP)	Idealists (NF)	Rationals (NT)
Myers-Briggs (MBTI types)	ESTJ, ISTJ ESFJ, ISFJ	ESTP, ISTP ESFP, ISFP	ENFP, INFP ENFJ, INFJ	ENTP, INTP ENTJ, INTJ
True Colors	Gold	Orange	Blue	Green
Diet Types	Diet Planners	Diet Players	Diet Feelers	Diet Thinkers

source of scientifically and nutritionally sound food facts presented in an easy-to-understand format that you can use in your day-to-day life. In The Basics, you'll learn the real facts about weight loss, exercise, and healthy eating. What you *won't* learn, is how to restrict entire food groups (there is nothing wrong with pasta and bread), how to live on wheat grass and beet juice (um, yuck and yuck) or how to steer clear of so-called "bad"

~ PERSONALITY 101

Want to learn even more on personality types and temperaments? Check out these entertaining and informative titles:
 Showing Our True Colors by Mary Miscisin
 Type Talk by Otto Kroeger
 Please Understand Me by David Keirsey
 Just Your Type and *Do What You Are* by Paul D. Tieger & Barbara Barron-Tieger

foods (chocolate and cheese taste too *good* to be ALL *bad*). As a registered dietitian *and* a food lover, I know the ins and outs of staying healthy and fit, *and* enjoying food! Even if you think you already have a solid nutrition knowledge base, read Chapter 7 for a refresher. Trust me here—you need this information if you want this book to work for you!

OK ladies, let's find your Diet Type and get started!

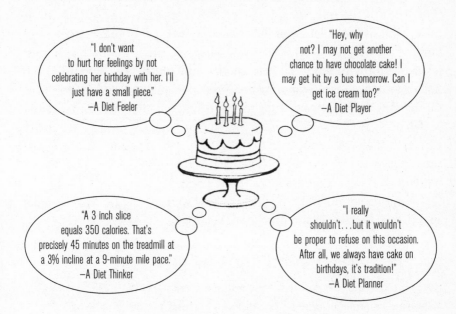

How the Diet Types Decide if They're Going to Have Birthday Cake

CHAPTER 2
Discovering Your Diet Type

Who Are You?

Finding your Diet Type is a little like a treasure hunt. You're looking for the hidden parts of your personality using a series of clues—in this case, the clues we use to unlock the "true you" are your answers to the following questions. But each question isn't a "yes" or a "no" question. Instead, the questions ask you to choose descriptions that best match your personality.

You will select descriptions from one personality category or the other, count them up, and whichever you have more of is your dominant trait. (For some of the questions, you may check off some descriptions from each columns for others, you may match up with all of one category and none of the other. That is OK! If you select qualities from both columns, just add up the number of check marks, and whichever column has the highest number represents your dominant personality trait.) As you read through the following four categories of different preferences and pick the preference you feel most reflects you, be sure to pick the characteristics you really do have, as opposed to the ones you want to have, or think you should have. Remember: no preference is better or worse than another, so just choose the one that describes you the best.

An important note: If you already know your four-letter MBTI® code, simply turn to page 13 and find your Diet Type.

DON'T BOX ME IN!

As you take the test, keep in mind that the personality theory is not about labeling or limiting individuals. After all, besides temperament, people's identity is shaped by age, experience, gender, cultural background, education, birth order, and many other factors. Nevertheless, understanding your temperament (and, in turn, your Diet Type) provides a glimpse at the "why" behind what you do (and don't do) and helps you identify not only what motivates you, but also what stresses you out. And because losing weight and keeping it off is a multi-dimensional process—physically, emotionally and psychologically—understanding yourself arms you with the necessary answers and insights you need for ultimate success. In short, no one knows "you" better than "you," and knowing who you are is the most important information you can have when it comes to losing weight, eating healthy, and changing your lifestyle—for life!

Question One: Where do you like to direct your time and energy?

Extraverts tend to be more open and social, focusing their time and efforts on the world around them. *Introverts*, on the other hand, turn most of their energy towards their own inner world, a world of their own thoughts and perceptions, and thus they tend to be more reserved and private.

Extraverts:
Are gregarious
Enjoy large groups
Are expressive
Act then think
Like to be where the action is
Think out loud

Are energized by being
  with people

Introverts:
Are reflective
Enjoy one-on-one social situations
Are reserved
Think then act
Focus on one thing at a time
Process thoughts internally on
  their own
Are energized by spending time
  alone

Are you an Extravert (E) ___ or an Introvert (I) ___

Question Two: How do you learn about life?

Sensors tend be interested in what is happening in the "here and now" and will often gather their information by observing and experiencing the world through their five senses. *Intuitives* are more interested in what could be, including future possibilities, and they gather information through instincts, perceived meanings, and correlations.

Sensors:
Are more interested in what is

Focus on the present; the here and
  now
Value common sense
Pay attention to specifics and details
Prefer facts and concrete information
Are realistic and pragmatic
Trust their experiences

Intuitives:
Are more interested in what is
  possible
Focus on the future; what might be

Value innovation
Pay attention to the big picture
Prefer insights and theories
Are inventive and inspired
Trust their hunches

Are you a Sensor (S) ___ or an Intuitive (N) ___
(Note: the letter N is used for intuitive because I is used for Introvert.)

Question Three: How do you make decisions?

Thinkers are objective (make decisions based on facts) and tend to analyze the problem first, and consider the people involved with the problem second. This is because they base decisions on logical reasoning. *Feelers* are subjective (make decisions based on personal beliefs) and tend to consider people involved with the problem first, and the problem second. This is because they base decisions on personal values.

Thinkers:
Analyze the problem
Are direct
Seek clarity
Problem 1st/People 2nd
Are objective
Are good at critiquing
Are firm-minded

Feelers:
Sympathize with peoples' problems
Are tactful
Seek harmony
People 1st/Problem 2nd
Are subjective
Are good at appreciating
Are fair-hearted

Are you a Thinker (T) ___ or a Feeler (F) ___

Question Four: How do you arrange your life?

Judgers like to have things decided in advance, prefer structure, and feel more comfortable controlling their environment. *Perceivers* don't want to miss anything, so they like to keep their options open at all times; they are also more comfortable adapting to their environment.

Judgers:
Value structure
Like to plan ahead
Will work now and play later
Would rather complete projects
Like order and neatness
Like to have decisions made
Are productive and organized

Perceivers:
Value flexibility
Plan as they go
Will play now and work later
Would rather start projects
Like randomness and adapting
Like to leave options open
Are spontaneous and often "play it by ear"

Are you a Judger (J) ___ or Perceiver (P) ___

Based on whichever preference you picked the most of for each question, fill in your four-letter code and find your Diet Type...

E or I   _____
S or N   _____
T or F   _____
J or P   _____

The Diet Planners
- ESTJ
- ISTJ
- ESFJ
- ISFJ

The Diet Players
- ESFP
- ISFP
- ESTP
- ISTP

The Diet Feelers
- ENFP
- INFP
- ENFJ
- INFJ

The Diet Thinkers
- ENTJ
- INTJ
- ENTP
- INTP

Who's Inside Your Head?*

With phrases that are designed to tap into some of the internal dialogue, diet reasoning, and weight loss wishes you might be experiencing every day, you may find that this exercise makes it easier for you to spot yourself. If the wording of the answers is not totally precise, that's OK; just pick what most closely resembles the way you think about you, eating, and losing weight.

1. Reasons I gained weight:

A   Overextended with work and home responsibilities; busy schedule; low priority.

B   Boredom; Impulse eater; I LOVE food!

C   Emotional eating; personal or relationship stress; low self-esteem.

D   Genetics (like slow metabolism), medication side effects, injury or illness.

2. Reasons I want to lose weight:

A   Better health, fit into my clothes again, it's the right thing to do.

B   More energy, look fantastic, participate in more activities.

C   Feel better about myself, improve my self-esteem, feel good emotionally and physically.

D   Decrease health risk factors like lower blood pressure, cholesterol... be more comfortable.

3. How I justify not managing my weight:

A   So many other responsibilities, I have picked up bad habits along the way that I have had a hard time breaking.

B   It's too much work, I'd rather enjoy my life right here, right now.

C   I am going through an emotionally tough time and food provides comfort. Others need me, I'd feel selfish putting my needs first.

D   There's no conclusive scientific evidence that being thin is actually healthy. I haven't found a formula that works for me yet.

* copyright 2009 by Mary Miscisin

4. When it comes to weight management:

A   Just tell me what to eat, how much to eat and when to eat it. I do well with schedules, routines and planning ahead.

B   I'm spontaneous and like to make quick decisions. I need to be able to make a healthy choice when the impulse hits me.

C   I prefer a holistic approach that addresses both mind and body. I like to eat food that feels good in my body and that I feel good about eating.

D   I like to have a system, developed by researching and devising an approach specific to my needs based on competent information sources and experience.

5. Things I would find helpful in a weight management approach:

A   Preparing ahead; having a plan and sticking to it; routines for maintaining a healthy lifestyle, being accountable.

B   Quick results; impulse control; flexibility, competition, a variety of physical activities; easy ways to grab a healthy bite to eat.

C   Support from others; sharing feelings, issues and ideas; journaling; self-development—finding my path/purpose; understanding that self-love is not selfish.

D   Information and resources regarding diet and exercise from competent sources so I can study independently.

If you picked mostly A's—you have the characteristics of a **Diet Planner**

If you picked mostly B's—you have the characteristics of a **Diet Player**

If you picked mostly C's—you have the characteristics of a **Diet Feeler**

If you picked mostly D's—you have the characteristics of a **Diet Thinker**

If you are tied for two on top—you are a combo Diet Type—read both

Will the Real You Please Step Forward...

Congratulations! You've found your Diet Type! You are already well on your way to success.

Before we get started, let's just take a little extra time to make sure that your Diet Type is really "clicking" with you...like anything else in life that is really important, we want to be sure it's "the real thing" before we start to make life changes.

Even though you were probably extra careful to choose qualities from the quiz that are most like you, pressure to change who we are is all around us—so much so, in fact, that even the most careful self-evaluation can be skewed by answers based on how you think you *should* be, rather than *how you really are*.

So, in the next step, we're going to take a look at the main characteristics of the Diet Types to make sure you have found your match.

As you read over the description of your Diet Type, ask yourself, "is this really me?" Be sure to go with your gut. In other words, you should get a "That is SO me!" feeling when you read about your Diet Type.

However, please be aware that, most likely, every single word or sentence in the descriptions below will *not* describe you completely—that is because you are unique, after all! But don't panic; as long as one Diet Type describes you more than the other three, you have found your Diet Type.

THE DIET PLANNERS ARE:

- ESTJ
- ISTJ
- ESFJ
- ISFJ

BEING A DIET PLANNER...

- I have a strong sense of what is right and wrong
- I take my duties and responsibilities seriously
- Home, family, and stability are important to me
- I am organized and hard working
- I like to feel useful and valuable
- Friends would consider me loyal and dependable
- I have a strong work ethic and expect the same from others

- I like to be prepared and tend to look before I leap
- I think discipline and teamwork are important for completing tasks
- I believe it is an honor to be elected to an office
- Fulfilling my personal and professional commitments means a lot to me
- I hope for the best, but prepare for the worst
- Thoroughness and attention to detail are important to me
- I respect authority and follow rules
- I am a natural helper and a giver

Sound like you? Then you must be a Diet Planner! The Diet Planner values security and stability. She works hard, follows the rules, and expects others to do the same. Self-disciplined and reliable, she wants to do the right thing and she likes being held accountable for her actions.

The Diet Planner relies on responsibilities and rules to guide her life and help her make decisions. When it comes to her health, the Diet Planner does best when she is organized and orderly and she thrives on weight loss plans that offer structure and routine. See page 25 for more on the Diet Planners.

THE DIET PLAYERS ARE:

- ESFP
- ISFP
- ESTP
- ISTP

BEING A DIET PLAYER...

- I believe today must be enjoyed, because you never know about tomorrow
- Skill and cleverness are important to me
- I seek fun, variety, stimulation and excitement
- I am resourceful, adventurous, and enjoy living in the moment
- I like to act on my impulses and tend to leap before I look
- I am energetic, spontaneous, and love a challenge
- In a crisis, I act quickly to solve the problem
- Friends would consider me exciting, happy, and fun-loving
- I feel stumbling blocks are only temporary
- I think rules should be adapted to suit the situation

- Waiting for something to happen is frustrating... I just want to get on with the show
- In a restrictive and confined environment, I get bored and restless
- I take pleasure in making an impression on others
- I regard life as a game, to be played in the here and now
- I am a natural trouble-shooter, performer, and competitor

Ring any bells? Chances are you're a Diet Player! The Diet Player values spontanaiety and immediate action. She trusts her impulses, doing what is needed to get the outcome she wants. Flexible and adaptable, the Diet Player enjoys living in the moment.

As for losing weight and changing her eating habits, the Diet Player values her freedom and flexibility above everything else. She doesn't like to be burdened by strict diet rules and regulations; instead, she needs workable lifestyle solutions for effective, long-term weight loss. See page 59 for more on Diet Players.

THE DIET FEELERS ARE:

- ENFP
- INFP
- ENFJ
- INFJ

BEING A DIET FEELER...

- I am interested in new ideas that relate to people
- I am concerned with personal growth and development
- Harmonious relationships are very important to me
- I am conscious of people's emotions and see potential in everyone
- I am an excellent communicator
- Friends would consider me idealistic, passionate, and optimistic
- I invest a lot of energy in my personal relationships
- I believe compassion and genuineness are essential for myself and others
- I think people should work together to achieve their goals
- I have a strong desire for peace and harmony
- It is important for me to find meaning in the way I use my time

- I'm good at negotiating and peacekeeping
- I don't like working with people who don't appreciate and encourage
- Identity and self-actualization are important to me
- I seek meaning and significance in my life

Can you relate? Then you are a Diet Feeler! The Diet Feeler values relationships and unity. Passionate and perceptive, she appreciates and inspires others, often acting as a teacher or counselor to friends, family, and colleagues. In addition, her own personal quest to find meaning in her life is very important to her.

To realize her weight loss desires, the Diet Feeler does best with a holistic approach—that is, when considering her mental, emotional, social, spiritual and physical well-being as interconnected aspects that each influence the other. Getting in touch with her own needs and values helps her put her most natural, heartfelt efforts towards her health, because she needs to understand how what she can do today will fulfill her visions of the future. The Diet Feeler excels in weight loss when her efforts focus on self-expression, and especially when she receives positive encouragement and support from others along the way. See page 99 for more on Diet Feelers.

THE DIET THINKERS ARE:

- ENTJ
- INTJ
- ENTP
- INTP

BEING A DIET THINKER...

- I seek knowledge and understanding
- Intelligence and competency are very important to me
- I tend to be skeptical and want logical answers for everything
- Friends would consider me independent and intellectual
- I enjoy finding new and different ways of doing things
- I am constantly evaluating my abilities and I am my own worst critic
- I feel compelled to master things that come my way

- I am capable of analyzing and understanding complex information
- I enjoy discussing and debating new theories and ideas
- I value rationality and objectivity
- I believe knowledge means power
- I enjoy being intellectually challenged
- I strive for achievement and success
- I expect people to live up to my high standards
- Efficiency and clear thinking are important to me
- I tend to focus on long-term goals and look mainly to the future

Is it all adding up? Your responses indicate you are a Diet Thinker! The Diet Thinker values knowledge and competence. She is a life-long learner who strives to understand the world. She is prone to ignoring things that she feels are not worthy of her time—including her health.

When it comes to eating well and losing weight, an effective way for the Diet Thinker to begin is by making her diet a priority. Then she can use her keen intelligence to help her succeed. The Diet Thinker needs comprehension and information to realize and maintain her weight loss and fitness goals. See page 159 for more on Diet Thinkers.

HELP! I CAN'T FIND "ME!"

What do you do if you don't get that "That is SO me!" feeling?

If you are still struggling to identify your Diet Type, consider taking the in-depth Myers Briggs Type Indicator (MBTI®).

The Association for Psychological Type (APT) can help you locate a trained professionals to administer the MBTI® assessment to you (www. aptcentral.org), or you can take the test online at www.mbticomplete.org . Although the MBTI® may take some time, keep in mind that the information you will gather about yourself can be useful to you in all areas of your life, not just weight loss.

WHAT IF YOU ARE A COMBO TYPE?

For some, a single Diet Type just doesn't tell the entire story. If you feel that you have strong, defining characteristics from more than one Diet Type, then you are most likely a Combo Type. But don't worry! There is a simple way to learn the specifics of your Combo Diet Type so you can use this book in a way that works best for you.

Go over the bulleted lists for all four Diet Types again and check off the items on the list that are most like you. Then, rank the Diet Types based on which Type has the most check marks. Finally, order those Types from the most like you, to least like you. This will give you your *Diet Type Spectrum*.

Take the Types that you have ranked as your first and second "most like you" types and use those to create your Combo Diet Type. Then read the chapter of your most dominant Diet Type first, then follow it up by reviewing the Diet Type that is second in line.

Of course, if you get the sense that the first two dominant Diet Types alone *still* don't paint the full picture of who you are, look over the chapters on the other Types and pick and choose strategies that fit you the best.

Remember: this book is a tool for *you* and nobody else, so feel free to use it in any way you need to!

SEX IN THE CITY DIET TYPE

In the HBO series and movie, *Sex and the City*, four successful, single women live, love, and date in The Big Apple. The four friends get together to swap stories, offer support, compare dating notes, and share their hopes and dreams. Stylish, sexy, and witty, it's hard not to fall in love with this show, and with the four very different women. If you think about it, each woman could represent one of the four Diet Types, and approach eating and dieting in the same unique way that she approaches dating:

Charlotte York has an old-fashioned, traditional attitude toward dating and men. Like any good Diet Planner, Charlotte longs for stability and security.

Samantha Jones is a fun-loving Diet Player who is always up for a good time. She lives and loves to the fullest and is looking for Mr. Right Now as opposed to Mr. Right.

Carrie Bradshaw is an incurable romantic who is constantly on the lookout for her ideal mate. She's an emotionally vulnerable and imaginative Diet Feeler.

Miranda Hobbes has a no-nonsense approach to men. Skeptical and analytical, she's a Diet Thinker trying to balance her career and her love life.

PART TWO

Your

Diet Type

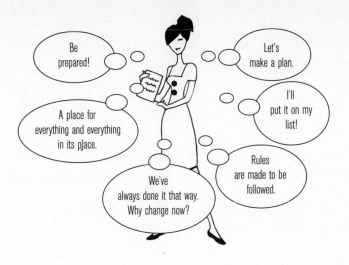

Inside a Diet Planner's Head

CHAPTER 3

The Diet Planners
ESFJ, ISFJ, ESTJ, ISTJ

In This Chapter...

THE DIET PLANNER PERSONALITY

- Likes to be Prepared
- Seeks Membership
- Organized
- Craves Consistency
- Penchant for the Past
- Divas of Detail
- Responsible
- Relies on Rules

THE DIET PLANNER TROUBLE SPOTS

- Eating Out of Character
- Not Prioritizing Your Health
- Forming Unhealthy Habits
- Being too Methodical
- Pessimistic about Outcome

THE DIET PLANNER SOLUTION

- How to Beat Your Trouble Spots
- The Diet Planner Plan

The Diet Planner Personality

Diet Planners are dependable, hard working, trustworthy, reliable and conscientious. They make loyal partners, responsible parents and solid leaders. Practical and down-to-earth, the Planners are concerned citizens who trust authority and seek security. They're the good-hearted and good-natured adherents of the tried and true.

> **Diet Planners of Fame and Fortune:** Martha Stewart, Barbara Walters, Queen Elizabeth II, and Mother Theresa all embody the characteristics of a Diet Planner.

Prepared and detail-oriented, you can always count on a Diet Planner. Have you ever seen the movie *The Wedding Planner* starring Jennifer Lopez? The opening scene makes it clear that Jennifer, a wedding planner, takes being prepared *very* seriously, especially on her client's "big day." In the frantic final moments before the trip down the aisle, Jennifer's character opens her jacket and reveals a hidden "emergency belt" containing everything from a sewing repair kit to breath mints, grooming products, and band aids. Hem of a bridesmaid gown coming down? She's got it covered with her handy needle and thread. Mother of the bride having a bad hair day? Not to worry, she'll fix her up with hairspray and a comb. Ring bearer scraped her knee? No problem, she'll whip out a band aid. In other words, you name a disaster... and like any good Diet Planner, she's prepared for it.

When a lady as buckled down as this planner takes on a weight loss plan, she operates with the same set of ideals she uses in every other area of her life. She wants to know that she has picked the right diet, that she is starting it at the right time, that she is going to work with the right people... in short, that she is going to be doing everything *right*! This attention to detail is one of many things that makes this amazing woman a classic Diet Planner.

> **Diet Planners in the Movies and on TV:** Charlotte from *Sex in the City*, Sally in *When Harry Met Sally*, and Monica on *Friends*.

Let's take a closer look at the Diet Planner's personality and examine how her core needs and motives influence her approach to a weight loss and diet program. Then, we'll take a look at the Diet Planners most common weight loss stressors and diet downfalls.

As you read through the following attributes of a typical Diet Planner, take the time to consider how, and to what extent, each personality trait applies to you and your life. Not all of the characteristics may match up with you—that's OK. This chapter is not supposed to limit you. Instead, the most important thing this chapter can do for you is help you get to know yourself. It is only through this process that you will *discover your personal weight loss challenges, and create a plan to use your personality strengths to achieve lasting, healthy weight success.*

DIET PLANNERS AT A GLANCE

Loyal to system	Decisive
Duty	Stability
Super dependable	Social responsibility
Preserves tradition	Structure
Precise	Orderly
Resists change	Authority dependent
Procedures	

Source: Otto Kroeger Associates www.typetalk.com

Likes to Be Prepared

" I plan ahead before going grocery shopping and I always shop with a list. I also like to plan what to eat for a whole day at a time, a week at a time is even better... that way I can be prepared.**"**
—JEANINE, A DIET PLANNER

There is a reason we call them Diet Planners... they LOVE to plan! Cautious and careful, Diet Planners like to be prepared for anything and everything. In fact, they like to have back-up plans for their back-up plans!

Diet Planners know that things can happen or come up—the unpredictable...the random...the sudden...and they want to make sure they will be able to handle any circumstance successfully.

Diet Planner's "prepare" to eat right by studying food labels, looking up nutrition information, planning meals, and getting the "facts" about foods and portions. Diet Planners don't mind breaking out the measuring cups or counting calories or points.

Seeks Membership

> **"** For weight loss success, group support is a big thing. **"**
> —JAN, A DIET PLANNER

Belonging to an organization, networking group, committee, family, community, club, etc. is one of the biggest pleasures of a Diet Planner and they'll work hard to protect the roles of everyone within the groups they support. They like to feel valuable and useful and derive satisfaction knowing they are contributing their fair share to the common good of the group. Loyal and faithful, they pay close attention to make sure everyone behaves in accordance with their membership privileges. Weight loss groups like Weight Watchers with clear rules and a community base work extremely well for the group-oriented, rule abiding Diet Planners.

Organized

> **"** I like to keep a detailed and organized log of my diet and
> exercise progress. **"**
> —STACIE, A DIET PLANNER

"A place for everything and everything in its place," is practically a Diet Planner's mantra! She likes to keep things clean, orderly and neat. The pantry of a proud Planner is a sight to behold...every can of vegetables is turned so the labels face out, and they might be arranged either alphabetically, by color, or by food group. Needless to say, disarray drives the Diet Planner crazy, and whether it's the dishes in the cupboard, the clothes in her closet, or the project she's working on, a Diet Planner has to finish what she started and put things back where they belong, before she can start her next endeavor. Notorious for making lists (and actually using them!) the Diet Planner derives a keen sense of satisfaction from crossing things off her "to do" list. When it comes to weight loss, the Diet Planner is most successful when she can put her organizational skills to good use.

Craves Consistency

> ❝ Breakfast and lunch are easy since I always have the same things, dinner is my challenge. ❞
> —ANNIE, A DIET PLANNER

Diet Planners like to arrange their lives so they know what to expect, and know exactly what's around every corner. Surprises are generally not enjoyable for a Diet Planner, who would rather experience the security of predictability rather than leave things to chance. For instance, Diet Planners like to eat on a schedule, rather than rely on hunger to signal them. If it is noon, it is time to eat lunch. Diet Planners enjoy habits and many have a set routine for how they start the day (wake up, turn on coffee, drink a glass of water and take a multi-vitamin, exercise, shower, eat yogurt and fruit, pack lunch, etc...). For this reason, it is key that a Diet Planner's weight loss routine fits easily into her structured way of life.

Penchant for the Past

> ❝ I want to go back to my past comfortable weight. I have loads of clothes in my wardrobe that don't fit me! ❞
> —HILARY, A DIET PLANNER

Traditionalists at heart, Diet Planners pay attention to the past and pay tribute to life's significant events. Celebrations, holidays and anniversaries are all cherished by Diet Planners, who love to orchestrate events down to the last detail. Family food traditions are ingrained into the life and blood of a Diet Planner. Grandma's famous baked beans at the Fourth of July, mom's to-die-for scalloped potatoes on Thanksgiving, chocolate cake on sister's birthday... the list goes on and on. Revamp grandma's bean recipe? A birthday without cake? Blasphemous!

When making decisions, Diet Planners look first to the past to established norms or what has worked before. That's why changing a family recipe, substituting a new dish for a traditional one, or breaking routine can be scary territory for the Diet Planner who likes things just the way they have always been.

Divas of Detail

> " I exercise on Mondays, Wednesdays and Fridays from
> 10:15 to 11AM, 7½ minutes of warm up, 30 minutes of
> aerobics and 7½ minutes of cool down. "
> —JAN, A DIET PLANNER

When it comes to specifics, these ladies don't miss a beat. If you ask what they had for breakfast, you won't get a simple reply, such as "Scrambled eggs." Instead, they'll give you all the details: "I had a 3-egg scramble with green pepper, sliced onion, sliced mushrooms and just a touch of butter." When ordering in a restaurant, Diet Planners want to make sure their server has all the details so they will get the order *just* the way they want it. For example, in the movie *When Harry Met Sally*, when Sally (played by Meg Ryan) eats out at a diner, her attention to detail/Diet Planner qualities are impossible to miss. She places her order like this: "I'd like the chef salad please with the oil and vinegar on the side and the apple pie a la mode. But I'd like the pie heated and I don't want the ice cream on top, I want it on the side, and I'd like strawberry instead of vanilla if you have it, if not then no ice cream just whipped cream, but only if it's real, if it's out of a can then nothing." In true Diet Planner fashion, she gets every detail exactly right.

Responsible

> **"** I am concerned about the long-term implications of being overweight and I would like to set a good example for my children and grand children. **"**
> —ANNIE, A DIET PLANNER

Conscientious and dependable, Diet Planners like to be held accountable. They take pride in a job well done and want to make sure it is not only done well, but also done on time. Diet Planners like to take on a lot of responsibility and they don't mind putting work before play so they can serve and do their duty.

Diet Planners are self-disciplined and dedicated, and they want to see tangible results for their efforts. They are also super-efficient and hate to waste anything. All that means that when a Diet Planner starts a weight loss program, she will work hard within expected guidelines to reach the goals she sets for herself.

Relies on Rules

> **"** I'm definitely a member of the clean plate club. **"**
> —JAN, A DIET PLANNER

Diet Planners like to follow the rules, use protocol and stick to procedure. They like to uphold the cultural norms of their Country, communities, workplace and home. It is tough for Diet Planners to just sit by and watch others break the rules.

They take the lessons their parents taught them to heart. Many Diet Planners were taught to clean their plate and feels she is "following the rules" by eating everything put in front of her. Besides, isn't it also rude to turn down a meal someone offers you or to be "picky"? A clear set of diet dos and don'ts is key for a Diet Planner, who likes to know what is expected of her at all times.

WHAT WORKS FOR DIET PLANNERS

Rules, routines and schedules
Weight loss meetings
Tracking progress
Short-term goals
Being accountable
Incentive planning

WHAT'S UP DOC?

Colleen's Story: A Diet Planner

“ Everything just happened so fast. We moved, the kids started school and my husband started a new job. I just don't have the energy to do anything anymore! **”**

Colleen took great pride in being a "traditional" stay-at-home mom. She had married her high school sweetheart at 21, bought a house just blocks from her parents, and worked hard at raising her three children and staying active in her community. Established routines for schoolwork time, dinner time and bedtime ensured that her household ran like clockwork, and Colleen kept her "dream house" meticulously clean. On top of her busy life at home, Colleen was also an active member of her church, the homeowners association, and a neighborhood book club. But all this changed when Colleen's husband was transferred to another state. Suddenly, Colleen found herself living in a different home and an unfamiliar community. Even the time zone was different!

This amount of change in such a short period of time would leave anyone feeling stressed and out of control. But to a Diet Planner like Colleen, a stable and secure external world is vital to a stable and secure inner world. So when so many things change so quickly, the results can be disastrous.

When Colleen showed up for her doctor's appointment, she looked and sounded very stressed out. Her appearance was a lot more disheveled than usual; I had never seen her with a loose ponytail or without make-up. I also noticed that she had gained weight. In fact, after her exam, I learned that she had gained more than 30 pounds in the past 6 months, and her blood pressure was now in the borderline risk range.

"I have these terrible headaches, and I can't even make the simplest decisions because I have trouble focusing," she told me, "and, to top it off, I can't fit into any of my old clothes! It's hopeless! I just don't have the energy to do anything anymore."

In the midst of uncertainty and confusion, Diet Planners need someone to help take control and prescribe a plan that they can follow. This helps them get back on their feet. This authority figure may come in the form of a coach, mentor, friend, religious leader, or any other person the Diet Planner holds in high regard. Today, as her physician, I was going to have to help guide Colleen.

"You must set a regular series of appointments to get your *life* and then your *health* back on track," I said. "And that's an order," I told her sternly, yet with a reassuring smile. I knew that I had to help Colleen establish structure in her external world so that she could feel internally grounded enough to deal with her health issues successfully. For a Diet Planner, attempting to address emotional issues like weight loss before they feel secure in their daily life would be futile.

With a set of appointments on her calendar, Colleen and I were now ready to tackle the specifics. At each one of our meetings, the two of us worked together on developing a comprehensive plan to help her regain structure in her life. First, we made a checklist of daily activities to help her get her home in order. Then, we addressed the need for new routines for the children. Once Colleen felt more in control, I gave her "assignments." These tasks would help Colleen focus on her emotional needs, like her need for a sense of belonging in her community. One "assignment" was for her to develop a relationship with her neighbors and investigate membership in local groups.

As the weeks and months went by and Colleen followed her "assignments" and her checklists, her vital sense of well-being in her internal and her external world were well established. This was the perfect time for us to focus on her health needs. We carved time into her schedule for regular exercise and made a list of everyday, healthy meals.

On our last appointment, Colleen reported that her headaches had disappeared, and her energy had returned. And on top of all that great news, Colleen's weight and blood pressure had dropped to a normal range. At last, with her world in order, she was in a place where she could take care of others—and guard her own health to ensure that she will be there for her family, friends and community for a long, long time.

—Dr. Redard

The Diet Planner Trouble Spots

Although there may be many different aspects to a Diet Planner's personality, her driving force is wanting to feel that she is in control at all times, and that she is following along with the rules the way she should be. This means that these loyal ladies require customs and rules to guide them, thrive in structured environments, and need duties to work towards.

All that being said, you can imagine why a Diet Planner has everything lined up for weight loss success! Most diets require preparation, and a tuned-in Diet Planner is primed and ready for anything. She'll carry nutritious snacks and a bottle of water wherever she goes. She'll schedule work outs and always remember to pack her gym shoes and clothes. She'll make food shopping lists, plan her meals, and schedule her indulgences.

Sounds like her success is guaranteed, right?

Well, the trouble is, regardless of how organized and prioritized her day may be, a Diet Planner—just like all of us!—simply cannot control everything. When "life gets in the way" the Diet Planner trips up. Below, we will take a look at how. We will also take a look at how a Diet Planner can anticipate her own weaknesses—and then nip them in the bud using her own strengths. But let's start with taking a look at the Diet Planner trouble spots.

Just as you did in the previous section, as you read through the following, take the time to consider how, and to what extent, each weakness may apply to you. And don't forget, even though you are one of many Diet Planners in the world, you are still totally unique, so you may not be able to relate to every example.

Eating out of Character

❝ When my life is out of control, so are my food choices. **❞**
　　—JAN, A DIET PLANNER

Under ideal circumstances, Diet Planners follow good eating habits to a "T." After all, as we saw in the first section, a Diet Planner relies on rules, and is an organized "Diva of Detail." But stressed-out Diet Planners who are pushed to their limits will morph from rule-abiding, balanced eating, calorie-counting Dr Jekyll's, into law-breaking, doughnut grabbing, over-eating Mr. Hyde's. For days, weeks, years, or even a lifetime, stress will throw the Diet Planner off. She'll toss aside her duty-bound goals, and she will "eat out of character," turning to high-calorie, unhealthy foods for comfort.

Work stress was the number one reason cited by Diet Planners for why they gained weight. It was not only that they themselves had so many responsibilities; they were also constantly taking up the slack of coworkers and taking on the work of others for the good of the organization (a Diet Planner wants to stick to the rules for the sake of the group, remember?). And to make matters worse, many of these dedicated ladies perceived they didn't get the appreciation they deserved for their efforts. This type of situation offers a stress (and dieting) double whammy for the Planner and can lead to out-of-control eating. So, instead of using food for nutrition and energy (a diet golden rule) they will turn to it for comfort and stress alleviation (a diet disaster).

Not Prioritizing Your Health

❝ My job is demanding and stressful and it leaves me little
　　time to work out and eat right. **❞**
　　　—STACIE, A DIET PLANNER

As someone who is powerfully productive and craves responsibility, Diet Planners tend to wear many hats—worker, spouse, friend, mother, caretaker, sister, event planner, community leader, PTA president, volunteer, etc. Therefore, it's no surprise that this Diet Type is often guilty of putting too much (literally and figuratively) on her plate. With so much to do, and so many people counting on her to make sure things get done, Diet Planners often find little time to take care of their own needs. In fact, a common weight loss Diet Planner complaint is "I'm too busy to lose weight."

Being responsible for their family, their work duties, and their social commitments may offer little, if any, time for their own "health obligations." And rather than say "no" to a perceived duty, under a great amount of stress, Diet Planners will often go into "responsibility overload," often becoming so rundown they catch a cold or the flu.

Forming Unhealthy Habits

❝ I eat out of routine and habit. I eat in front of the TV
   at night.**❞**
   —HILARY, A DIET PLANNER

Habits are an integral part of a Diet Planner's life. After all, she craves consistency, and has a penchant for the past. She loves comfortable and familiar structure. This Type will shop at the same grocery stores, buy the same foods, prepare the same recipes, eat at the same restaurants, and order the same foods, over and over and again.

All that is well and good... unless she's a Diet Planner with a weight problem. Then it's highly likely she's developed some rather unhealthy habits, like eating while watching TV or skipping breakfast. Diet Planners are predisposed to routine so they automatically want to continue their habits—good or bad. Diet Planners also tend to have a pessimistic view toward their weight troubles (see "Pessimistic About Outcome," below), and, combined with a need for consistency, many Diet Planners will *make weight loss failure a habit* just so they can keep things predictable. This intense desire to maintain a comfort zone—or should I say "un-comfort zone"—compels Diet Planners to hang on to bad eating and exercise habits longer than is healthy for them.

Habits from long ago can also come back to haunt the Diet Planner, because she is often nostalgic for the past. If a Diet Planner remembers how full-fat macaroni and cheese and a trip to the ice cream shop comforted her when she was a girl, she will turn to those foods again and again for stress management.

Being too Methodical

> " If I can't follow my diet perfectly, I'll give up on the entire
> thing."
> —JUDY, A DIET PLANNER

Just about every aspect of the Diet Planner's personality craves rules, routines and schedules. They are what help her be prepared, productive and responsible, as well as organized and consistent with the past. She loves details and rules, so keeping to a system comes naturally to her. And when it comes to weight loss, that can be a really, really good thing. However, life does not always run as smoothly as she'd like, and bumps in the weight loss road (and there are plenty of them!) can throw everything off course, leading to frustration, disappointment, and, if she is not careful, failure.

An unscheduled meeting, a sick child, a broken appliance—these events typically set in motion an instantaneous re-scheduling, re-organization, and re-prioritizing of the day. This is all to keep the Diet Planner on track with her master task list. The problem is that, when things get rescheduled, many Diet Planners give highest priority to social/work obligations (external structure) than to personal health (internal structure). If the Diet Planner was able to fend off panic, set aside her task list, and leave some items to be wrapped up the next day, she would have an easier time putting her health first. Unfortunately, her commitment to a plan, above everything else, often prevents this from happening.

Pessimistic about Outcome

> " I have accepted that I will always struggle to keep my
> weight under control."
> — ANNIE, A DIET PLANNER

In lots of ways, a Diet Planner is a step ahead when it comes to dieting: she has the superior organizational skills needed to plan meals, keep track of intake, and schedule exercise, and her consistent, hard-working nature is ideal for staying the course. She likes routine, she'll follow reasonable rules, and once she builds healthy habits—she'll stick with them, forever.

Still, regardless of all her many, many weight loss advantages, it is in fact the Diet Planners who are the least optimistic about their chances for success. Why?

Well, because Diet Planners sensibly look to the past for direction in their present, if they have had unsuccessful weight loss attempts before, they will doubt that they can produce different results another time round. And, if they have never attempted to lose weight in the past, then they won't have any experiences (good or bad) to draw from for guidance—which means that, while they will hope for the best, they will be prepared for the worst. Also, because Diet Planners live in the here and now, they have trouble imagining a different future, even one where they are more healthy.

WHAT DOESN'T WORK FOR DIET PLANNERS

Tons of choices
Last-minute solutions
Processing without tangible results
Playing it by ear
Studying diet theories
Not having a solid plan

WHAT'S UP DOC?

Margaret's Story

**❝ I have been waiting for one hour and ten minutes!
This is unacceptable, doctor! ❞**

On first impressions Margaret appears to be in charge—self confident, assertive, and forthright with her opinions and rules for behaving.

"You're late!"

"I know Margaret, I'm sorry," I said rushing into the exam room.

"I had an appointment at two o'clock. It is now..." she lifted her hand and pointed to her watch, "Three ten. I have been waiting for one hour and ten minutes! This is unacceptable! Two o'clock means two o'clock. It doesn't mean two-ten, two-thirty, three, and most definitely it doesn't mean three-ten!"

For the past five years Margaret would make and keep her medical appointments. The first few minutes were usually spent discussing the way things *should* be, that is, the way that Margaret thinks they should be. Perhaps the weather is too cold, somebody cut her off in traffic, her co-workers are not doing the job they are supposed to, her supervisor is not giving her the direction she needs, her husband doesn't stack the dishes correctly, her children are not wearing the right clothes…the list is seemingly endless. Then she would finally give a detailed explanation of all her various ailments, aches, and pains which we would address one at a time.

At 5 foot 4 inches and 210 pounds her weight was a sizable problem. Margaret would follow a diet religiously and lose 20 or 30 pounds, and then there would be a "crisis" at work or home and she would revert to old habits and regain the weight. This pattern repeated itself again and again…until one particular appointment.

Margaret was not her usual confident, assured self—she seemed somehow beaten, deflated, and pre-occupied. When I asked how she was, she responded out of her usual character.

"I'm fine! I'm fine! The words spit out of her with such intensity that I could tell there was something else going on beneath.

"I guarantee you that you will feel much better if you tell me what is *really* going on," I responded.

"What do you mean?" she said appearing frightened.

I have seen this pattern again and again with Diet Planners–and I was almost certain that it was going on with Margaret too. We had five years invested in this relationship; if she wasn't going to trust me now she never would. It was time to get the cat out of the bag.

"*I've done a horrible thing!*" she finally confessed.

She had been married to her husband, Tom, for twenty years now. But three days before her wedding Margaret had a "fling." Although it was a one-time thing, it broke every rule and value that she held dear. The guilt and shame she felt year after year was nearly unbearable. And her weight reflected this.

After she was married she began to gain weight. Each time she had been slightly successful in weight loss, her anxieties rose (along with libido) and this terrified her. Her weight would rebound until she felt "safe" again. She experienced what many Diet Planners relate: a sense that they are "split in two"—a part that struggles to "do the right thing" and a secret part that desires or does what it condemns in others. In order to resolve Margaret's internal conflicts, and achieve long-term practical weight management, she would need to release the guilt and bring closure to her past.

For Diet Planners, rituals and ceremonies are important; measuring transition from one segment of life into another; Birthdays, Graduation, Weddings…Unfortunately, for unfinished business such as this, there are no culturally defined rituals—so we would have to devise one.

I suggested a letter-writing exercise. Although she never intended to send them, Margaret wrote letters to her husband admitting her actions and asking for forgiveness. Simply writing these letters were enormously soul-cleansing for her. One night when she had the house to herself, she sat in front of the fireplace with her letters and read each aloud, said a little prayer, and then threw them in the fire.

Also we worked on accepting shortcomings, hers as well as others. To simply observe that she might have the "right way" of doing things did not necessarily mean that she had to share this with the world. This is an exercise that she continues to practice daily.

With the guilt from her past resolved and her life back in balance, we could finally focus on Margaret's long-term practical weight loss approach.

She went to our staff nutritionist and got back on a reduced-calorie plan. Margaret has lost over 70 pounds and continues to make progress. She relates that she feels "safe" at her weight and no longer rebounds during "crisis." Her relationships with her co-workers and family have improved, and her relationship with her husband Tom is "solid."

I occasionally run late for her appointments, but since that day she has not said a word…

—Dr. Redard

The Diet Planner Solution

Part One of Your Solution:
How to Beat Your Trouble Spots

Now, let's take a closer look at some tips tailored to the Diet Planner personality that will help eliminate trouble spots. Finding a way to surmount trouble spots goes hand-in-hand with developing important life strategies that will work with who you are.

Read through the following Planner-friendly strategies for addressing key trouble spots, and decide if some (or all) of these things need to be addressed in your own life. Then, work through the advice, one solution at a time.

Here's a reminder of the Diet Planner's weaknesses:

- Eating Out of Character
- Not Prioritizing Your Health
- Forming Unhealthy Habits
- Being too Methodical
- Pessimistic about Outcome

How does a Diet Planner beat the tendency to "eat out of character?"
If stress is turning you into an out-of-control Mr. Hyde (you know who you are!), it's time to take a step back and uncover the *real* source of your anxiety.

~ FIRST STEPS TO SUCCESS

- Honestly examine your life to uncover the real source of your stress.
- Directly confront the problems in your life instead of turning to food for comfort or escape (see page 119 for more on emotional eating).

FIND THE SOURCE OF YOUR STRESS

Stress is simply the emotional and physical impact we experience when our basic psychological needs are not met. Although most people assume their needs are the same as every other human being, the truth is, different people have different needs. As a Diet Planner, for example, your need to feel in control and know that you are following the rules, are quite unlike the needs of a Diet Player (they crave the freedom to act in the moment and avoid rules at all costs!) Consciously and unconsciously, people seek to fulfill their basics needs, and if those needs are not being met, it leads to that great dieting downfall: stress.

So the big question is: are your Diet Planner needs being met?

Here are some things to ask yourself that will help you ascertain if the Diet Planner in you is satisfied, or if some aspects of your life are making you feel short-changed...

Are you a useful and practical part of a community, family, or group?

Is your life arranged in an orderly and scheduled manner?

At work, are your performance expectations clear to you? Do you receive useful feedback?

Do you feel that you are appreciated for your hard work and contributions, at work, at home, and anywhere else you are involved?

Do you feel that you are fulfilling your commitments and acting responsibly and dutifully?

Do you sense that an unsettling change in your life or routine may have propelled you into an unhealthy rut? (see Colleen's story page 32)?

Do you think you might have an unresolved issue from your past that needs to be addressed before you can focus on losing weight (see Margaret's story page 38)?

Hopefully, answering these questions has made you more aware of your core needs, and given you a sense of how they may or may not be addressed in your life right now. In this way, you will gain the insight needed to not only uncover the source of your stress, but also point you in the direction of personal satisfaction. I'm not saying it's possible to rid your life of *all* stress, (morning traffic, family pressures and work deadlines are not just

～ DIET PLANNER "TO DO" LIST

As a Diet Planner, you probably love checking items off your "to-do" list. Here is a list to get you started... and the best part is, you can *already* check everything off!

- **Learn more about myself and my weight loss weak spots so I can be prepared when I face a sticky (or sticky bun) situation.** Check! Reading the rest of this chapter and exploring your trouble spots will help you deal with the unexpected, make positive lifestyle changes, and prepare you to start your Diet Planner Plan.

- **Find a weight loss program that will not only help me lose weight, but also teach me how to keep it off for good.** Check! On page 53 you'll find your Diet Planner Plan with clear, step-by-step instructions. This plan takes advantage of all your Diet Planner strengths

- **Learn the basics of nutrition, weight loss and health from a reliable, credible source.** Check! In Chapter 7 you'll find a trustworthy source of nutritionally sound weight loss facts that are easy-to-understand. You'll learn the real specifics about healthy living, and discover why the benefits of weight loss go far beyond fitting back into your skinny jeans.

- **Find easy and healthy go-to meals I can turn to again and again.** Check! In Chapter 8 you'll find loads of delicious and nutritious meals created by registered dietitian and trained chef Tamara Goldis. You'll also learn how to create meals using your own favorite foods and recipes.

gonna disappear!), but meeting your basic core needs will give you a leg up when it comes to dealing with life's rough patches, and help you avoid the kind of "I am so overwhelmed!" stress that leads to serious self-destructive behaviors—like overeating.

For the Diet Planner who tends to put herself last, I cannot overemphasize that *it is your responsibility to ensure that your own needs are being met*, and you can't get healthy, eat well, and be successful at long-term weight loss—and help others—until you do. Although it may be hard at first, in the end there is no shortcut to fulfillment, and no substitute for, taking a long hard look at your life.

How does a Diet Planner make her own health a priority?

As a Diet Planner, how do you shift your priorities and take responsibility for your health, without feeling like your "to do" list is going to be compromised? Take a look at a successful endeavor from your past to help remind you that—lo and behold!—you have in fact been able to move priorities on your "to do" list around and not only survived... but succeeded! A shift in priorities can be scary, but it is essential if you want to shake those extra pounds.

～ FIRST STEPS TO SUCCESS

- Think back to a past accomplished goal and make the choice to use the same mind-set and determination needed to achieve your weight loss and health goals.
- When you are ready, sign a weight loss contract between yourself and an authority figure—a person you can report back to on your progress.

REALIZE YOUR RESPONSIBILITY

When you make something a priority it takes on a powerful significance and becomes a very important part of your life. As a Diet Planner, you most likely prioritize the needs of others, your work commitments, and your community duties, way above your own health needs. This means that, inevitably losing weight tends to get pushed to the bottom of your "to do" list. So, even though you *want* to lose weight, and even though you possess many in-born skills that would *help* you lose weight, in order to succeed you must make your health an important "duty."

So how do you adjust your viewpoint so you can re-order the items on your to do list a little bit?

Let's take a look at a little medical reality. In the short-term, your extra pounds might mean a larger pants size, some guilty feelings, and a self-imposed beach ban—disappointing, but certainly not devastating. However, in the long-term, your extra weight could mean diabetes, high blood pressure, a heart attack, and a shortened life span (gulp!). Now that's a serious and indeed very distressing state of affairs that fortunately, can be avoided altogether. Don't wait until a health emergency forces you to make your weight loss a priority. It's like not paying a bill until it is in collections. Or not putting oil in your car until it breaks down. Things you would *never* do!

The simple fact is, the world needs you to be in tip-top shape! Your Diet Type makes up 40 percent of the population, and Diet Planners contribute to the backbone of society... you gals are the world leaders, role models, and mentors. How can you be counted on to fulfill your responsibilities, help your community, and guide others if your weight is off the scales and your health is suffering? The answer is, you can't! So no more excuses—it's time to take care of yourself, and make guarding your health the "#1" item on your list of things to do.

How do I know this will work? Well, instead of looking into a crystal ball to get a glimpse of your future success... let's take a look at your past.

Look to the Past

Think back to one of your proudest accomplishments, be it starting a family, changing careers, graduating from college, organizing a fundraiser, finding a job, etc. Remember how hard you worked, and the time, energy, and commitment you employed to reach your goals?

Although it may not be obvious at first, you successfully re-arranged your life in order to make attaining those goals a possibility.

This same type of re-prioritizing is an important part of your dedication and commitment to a healthy lifestyle, and it is essential in order for you to meet your weight loss goal. Once you, Diet Planner extraordinaire, decide that your health is an important "must," and that you will have to reorganize your to-do list in order to reach that goal, you will be well on the way to success.

Bonus: as long as you are "back in the past," take a minute to examine what did and did not work for you if you tried to lose weight before. What lessons did you learn? Use these lessons as information to help you plan more wisely this time. Once again... *you* hold the key to paving your bright, healthy future!

Sign a Contract

When you are ready to make weight loss a priority, sign a contract with yourself and with someone else and enter your contract in your weight loss log (see page 54). Setting a contract with someone else helps keep you on track, makes you responsible, and provides you accountability and support. Your doctor is always a good choice, as is a dietitian or other health professionals. While a friend, or even your partner, will work too, it's best to pick an authority figure—a person you can report back to on your progress. Your contract can be as simple as a few lines, listing your ultimate goals (like losing 30 pounds), or it can be a detailed list of all the things you plan to do to lose the weight and keep it off.

How does a Diet Planner break unhealthy habits?

It's easier than you might think! Simply follow this 3-step process: recognize, record and replace.

～ FIRST STEPS TO SUCCESS

- Take the time to Recognize, Record and Replace your unhealthy habits.
- Transform one bad habit into a healthy one, once a week, until you have successfully transitioned your routine. If you want to tackle one habit, once a month, or one every few days, that works too. The important thing is that you make a plan, select a time frame, and stick with it.

Step One: Recognize Unhealthy Habits

An important part of breaking unhealthy habits is first to recognize what they are. You are unique, and your personal bad habits probably won't be the same as your neighbors, your friends, or even your spouse's, but, since you are a Planner, keep your eye out for these common Planner pitfalls:

- **Mindless eating**—munching while watching TV, snacking while surfing the net, nibbling while you prepare food, grabbing a handful of goodies every time you pass the reception desk...Diet Planners are prone to this kind of bad snacking because these little bites are able to pass "under the radar"—that is, they don't register in the Diet Planner's mind as being all that bad, since they are spontaneous and momentary. But all these "mindless" calories add up—and often end up—on your waist and hips. Not good! As a Diet Planner, remind yourself that the best, most civilized place to eat is at a table without distractions, and the best reason to eat is only because you are hungry. In short, always be mindful of what, when and why you are eating.

- **Cleaning your plate**—eating the entire portion of whatever you are served often means eating more than you really need to satisfy your hunger. Contrary to what the rule-aware Diet Planner might think, it is not rude, unacceptable or inappropriate to leave food on your plate. In fact, the queen of manners, Emily Post, says, it is A-OK to leave some food on your plate! In fact, she even says it's rather rude to clean your plate so thoroughly that it looks like you haven't eaten in days.

- **Not drinking enough water**—if you're thirsty, you're dehydrated. And thirst and dehydration are bad news: not only does dehydration make you tired, but thirst is sometimes mistaken for hunger (not just by Planners, but by all Diet Types). Filling up on aqua is an important part of your weight loss arsenal. Try to get at least 8 to 10 glasses a day. Never forget: your body needs water, and a lot of it.

- **Addicted to dessert**—Diet Planners have a penchant for the past… and if dinner at home just wasn't dinner without dessert, than this dangerous habit can carry over into adulthood. Make a change and switch from baked goods and other calorie-laden sweet treats to nutritious and delicious fruit, or other not-so damaging choices (see page 262). If you still crave that slice of pie or cake, at least try to make fruit the sole item on the dessert menu more often than not—and, if you are a guest and not given a choice of desserts, eat just a few bites of the decadent creation.

- **Skipping meals**—Busy Diet Planners often end up skipping meals in order to fit everything into their schedule. This is a big no-no! Missing meals leads to a slowed metabolism, and overeating later in the day. And there is another reason your Mom always told you to eat breakfast: it's a proven fact that people who eat breakfast (the most commonly skipped meal) are more successful at weight loss than those who skip.

- **Drinking your calories**—Juice, coffee drinks, sports drinks, vitamin water, soda, smoothies, and cocktails. Calories are hiding in your drinks. It's better for everyone to eat, not drink, their calories (see page 212).

- **Eating to alleviate stress**—Diet Planners are notorious for eating when they're stressed. But turning to food instead of dealing with the issue is a sure-fire way to pack on the pounds (see Eating Out of Character page 35).

STEP TWO: RECORD

Next, take a week to identify the unhealthy habits in your own life and record them in your weight loss log (see page 54). Be sure to take the time to examine these habits carefully. Putting your habits in writing for a week, and giving them such careful consideration, will not only make you more conscious of your bad habits, but will also help you understand the negative effect that these bad habits are having on your life. This is the key to finding the motivation to change. (Note: if you had an atypical week, or if you were unconsciously on your "best behavior" because you were recording your habits, record another week—or two or three—until you have regularity, and an accurate portrait of your life.)

STEP THREE: REPLACE

Once you realize what your bad health habits are, how often you are engaging in them, and what negative effect they have on your life, the next step is to find a healthy permanent replacement for the bad habits. Make a list of possible replacement behaviors for each recorded bad habit. Example: if your bad habit is skipping breakfast, possible replacement behaviors could include: waking up earlier so you have time to eat, grabbing a high-fiber bar and a piece of fruit on the way out the door, or finding some healthy options from a local take-out spot that you can pick up on the commute to work. Next, test out each option until you find the one that sticks! The goal is to transform bad habits into good ones, tackling them one a time, as frequently as you can.

How does a Diet Planner keep from being too methodical?

Striving to be the best you can be and working hard to meet your goals is a good thing! But when you are trying to lose weight, you need to accept that mistakes will be made in order for lessons to be learned and permanent changes to take place. This can be really hard for the high-achieving Diet Planner! Weight loss and successful eating takes time, patience and the ability to give yourself a break every now and again. How does a Diet Planner accomplish this, when she is so committed to routine?

~ FIRST STEPS TO SUCCESS

- Realize that diet and exercise slip-ups are inevitable, and instead of striving for perfection, strive to learn from your mistakes and to change your lifestyle permanently.
- Set yourself up by always being prepared for the unexpected.

PASS ON PERFECTION

Improving your health, enhancing your lifestyle, and losing weight all mean *making a change*, and just like anything new (a new job, a new city, a new boyfriend) there are bound to be challenges. Some days, things will go your way and you'll do everything "right," but other days, unexpected problems and temptations are sure to come up, meaning that mistakes or slip-ups are inevitable. The thing is, if you are making mistakes, you are trying, and if you are trying you are learning. Much more important than always following the weight loss rules flawlessly, or always eating exactly the right foods, or always being "perfect" with your diet and activity, is *sticking with your plan*. Even if you have an off day, week, or (gulp!) month, don't stop! Keep going. In fact, the only difference between a Diet Planner that succeeds at weight loss and one that that fails, is that the winners don't give up. Instead, they learn from their mistakes, adjust their systems accordingly, and keep going. For example, if you over consume, calculate how much more exercise you need to do to make up for it, or figure out how much less you will have to eat over the next few meals to minimize the damage. Also, figuring out what happened will help you plan ahead so you are more prepared next time. And be sure to moderate, not eliminate... see below.

MODERATE INSTEAD OF ELIMINATE

Lots of Diet Planners assume that weight loss requires a diet of only "good" foods with complete avoidance of so-called "bad" foods. However, research shows that people with this "all or nothing" attitude tend to cycle between alternately dieting, and bingeing on their restricted foods. How to avoid this perilous pattern? The key is to follow a healthful eating plan, which focuses on whole grains, vegetables and fruits, lean protein choices and beans most of the time, and to *moderate* (that means carefully watch the amount of) rather than totally eliminate other not-so-healthy picks. You won't gain weight if you only *occasionally* indulge in high-fat, high-sugar, and high calorie foods. If you are sensible (hello—you are good at that!) and enjoy eating without overdoing it, you'll see results faster than by imposing harsh restrictions and setting yourself up to break your own rules.

PLAN TO BE PREPARED

Although your Diet Type has to be careful of being too hard on yourself and of getting frustrated when things don't go as planned, that's no reason not to set yourself up for success. In fact, just like the boy scouts, a Diet Planner's best defense against the unexpected is to be prepared, and it's no different with weight loss. Here's how...

- **Prepare to eat**—follow a reduced-calorie structured eating plan with clear rules and planned meals. Planning a week of menus at a time makes grocery shopping easier, and since your Diet Type doesn't mind eating the same foods, consider making large portions of favorite recipes to have on hand throughout the week.

- **Prepare for food risk occasions**—whether it's a birthday party, business conference, or friendly get-together, some person or food will try to tempt you to stray from your eating plan. Plan for it, rehearse what you will say and do ahead of time and execute your plan when the time arrives. For example, on the day of a birthday party plan to have a light breakfast and lunch, and to have just a small piece of cake at the party.

If you know the host is a "food pusher," come armed with a few reasons for insisting on a small piece. You can try saying, "no thank you, I had a huge lunch."

- **Prepare for activity**—It is imperative you make exercise a must, so schedule exercise as seriously as work or social appointments. Exercise classes that require reservations and scheduling (spinning, Pilates, or step aerobics, for example) are ideal for the Diet Planner. After all, you wouldn't be irresponsible and not show up for an appointment, would you?

- **Prepare for missed work outs**—a late meeting, an unexpected visitor, a sick child, whatever "it" is, always assume "it" will happen, and have a back up work out plan in place for when it does. So if you plan to go to a 6 PM spinning class, make your back up plan the 6 AM spinning class the next morning, saving a space in both classes just in case. You may not use your back-up very often, but as your Diet Type knows too well, it's better to be safe then sorry.

- **Prepare to indulge**—no need to completely give up your favorite not-so-healthy treats—just plan ahead. For example, plan a light breakfast and lunch on the day of an important evening event involving eating. Or save up your Craving Tamers (see page 262) for the week, and indulge in a special favorite dessert at the end of week.

- **Prepare for missed meals**—keep a stash of healthy snacks in your purse, gym bag, office and car in case of a missed meal emergency. If you keep your body consistently fed and satisfied, you will be less likely to stop at McDonald's, Krispy Kreme, or any other tempting fast-food joint.

- **Prepare to eat out**—when you know ahead of time where you will be dining, look online for a menu and nutrition facts (or call the restaurant to have a menu faxed), and then based on the info in the Restaurant Rundown, page 235, select better-for-you options before you get to the restaurant. Also, gather nutrition brochures from your regular spots and test out healthier options so you have a weight reducing- selection of picks you can turn to again and again.

How does a Diet Planner beat their pessimistic streak?

What's the secret to losing that pessimism? Simply put, Diet Planners need to release their grip on the past. Just because you have had trouble making a change to your eating habits in the past doesn't mean that you can't reach your goal. The key is for the Diet Planner to feel confident that the plan she has chosen is the "right" one that will guide her in times of difficulty. Of course, every Diet Planner needs to believe whole-heartedly that she has the power to make a permanent change. But she also needs the right tools to keep her on track. Lucky for you, you have just what you need! That's where the final ingredient comes in... your very own personal Diet Planner *Plan*!

⌇ FIRST STEPS TO SUCCESS

- Remember that success isn't achieved by half efforts. Commit to reaching your goals and follow every step of the guidelines in your Diet Planner Plan meticulously.
- Use your Diet Planner superior organizational skills needed to plan your meals, schedule your exercise, and build healthy habits for a lifetime.

REALIZE YOU HAVE THE RIGHT MIND-SET

By now, you've learned how important the right attitude is. Well, guess what? If you read Part One of the solution and took the time to gain a deeper understanding of yourself, your needs, your strengths, and your weaknesses then you've got the mindset that you need for success! You are prepared to face obstacles, and make changes in your life if necessary. You, are primed to succeed. All you need now is the right plan.

REALIZE YOU HAVE THE RIGHT PLAN

Diet Planners in particular need a plan that they know will work for them. Sensible and result-oriented, the Planner isn't going to stick with something if it's not working for her. She needs to feel confident in her weight loss plan and see results, in order to stick with it. So the trick is to find the RIGHT plan. One you can rely on, one that has been tested, one that draws on your natural strengths and one that is designed by a credentialed expert... and lucky for you The Diet Planner Plan below, is just that plan. It offers you the structure and rules you need to thrive, while still allowing you control of your choices and your life. It doesn't make you cut out all your favorite foods or toss out all your food traditions, and it is based on facts. It is a solid approach to help you structure your life in a way that will facilitate long-lasting weight loss. It is not a diet you go "on" or "off" but a *lifestyle approach* that incorporates permanent healthy behaviors into your lifestyle.

Part Two of Your Solution: The Diet Planner Plan

This plan is uniquely catered to your personality traits, and takes advantage of your superior organizational skills and your uncanny ability to schedule and manage your life efficiently.

Remember, this strategy *starts with you*—not with a diet. That means that you will enjoy eating well and exercising, because you will be acting according to a plan with clearly defined rules, and tracking your progress will help keep you motivated.

And by drawing on your inborn Diet Planner strengths you'll not only lose weight, you'll learn how to keep it off! So let's get started!

The Diet Planner Plan At-A-Glance
The best way for a Diet Planner to slim down and shape up is by taking it one sensible step at a time:

Step One: Prepare to Lose Weight
Step Two: Plan Your Weeks
Step Three: Chart Your Action
Step Four: Assess Your Progress
Step Five: Start Your Maintenance Plan

Step One: Prepare to Lose Weight

Get Informed—With so much conflicting nutrition and diet advice floating around it's difficult for the Planners (along with the Players, the Feelers and the Thinkers) to separate weight loss right from wrong. And to get it right (IT being weight loss, weight maintenance, and sustaining a healthy lifestyle) you have to know the right facts. Chapter 7 is a source of nutritionally sound weight loss facts you can trust, and once you get the inside scoop you'll be in a much better position to identify what's causing the harm (not to mention the weight gain) in your own life, and to make informed decisions about your health and well being. So before you do anything else, read Chapter 7—a few times.

Get a Weight Loss Log—Purchase a standard-size three-ring binder along with a three-hole punch so you can add and subtract pages to and from your log as need be. You will use this log to arrange your meals, record your goals, track your progress, and to make lists and action plans to help you deal with your trouble spots. Even once you reach your weight loss goal, you can continue to use this log to help you plan your meals and your weeks (see Start Your Maintenance Plan on page 56). Be sure you record your starting weight in the log at this time.

Step Two: Plan Your Weeks

Plan Your Goals—Considering your Diet Type has a tendency to get impatient when things take too much time, and considering the number one reason women throw in the weight loss towel is because they get fed up when they don't lose weight as fast as they thought they would, it's very important for you set realistic short-term weight loss goals. Achieving your short-term goals will have a positive impact on your health (and your state of mind), and it will help you reach your long-term target weight, one controllable step at a time.

Following the advice in Part Four of Chapter 7 (page 231), determine your first short-term goal (5 percent of your current weight) as well as the approximate amount of time it will take you to reach that goal (expect an average loss of about two pounds per week), and record this in your weight loss log. (Note: After you reach your first short-term goal, you just set a new short-term goal using the same formula, as many times as needed until you reach your ultimate long-term goal.)

Plan Your Weeks—The meals in Chapter 8 make it easy for you to plan meals and choose foods that deliver a healthy, delicious and weight loss inducing daily 1,550 calories, plus an extra 100 calories for optional Craving Tamers. (Craving Tamers allow you to keep all your favorite foods in your life by simply slimming down the portions.) Each breakfast meal has about 400 calories, each lunch has 450, each dinner has 550, each calcium-rich snack has 150 calories, and each optional Craving Tamers has 100 calories. All you have to do is pick from the meals provided, or create your own meals using your own favorite foods and recipes using the easy guidance provided. There are meal options for carb-lovers and protein-lovers alike.

Select a "planning" day one day of the week, and using your weight loss log, plan your meals and schedule your activity for a seven day time period. Try to plan all your meals, including the meals you think you will eat away from home, and also plan for the times and places you will exercise. Try to anticipate where eating and exercising conflicts may arise, a late business meeting or a party, for example, and have options ready. On your planning day, also prepare your shopping list, and then go grocery shopping.

Plan Your Rewards—Losing weight is hard work and it's important to recognize milestones along the way with non-food awards. And not just weight loss milestones, but also changing behaviors—like giving up soda, attending weight loss meetings, or going to the gym. On the same day of the week that you plan your meals and activity, also determine your weekly goals and the incentives you feel are appropriate rewards for accomplishing those goals, like a CD or a manicure for not missing a scheduled work out all week or a pair of shoes for reaching your first short-term weight goal. Save bigger rewards (such as a vacation or a piece of jewelry you've had your eye on) for when you reach your long-term goals. The best reward for you is simply whatever will help you stay motivated, focused, and raise your awareness of what you've accomplished.

Step Three: Chart Your Action

Charting your daily action will help you understand when or if your health plan goes awry. Take time at the end of each day (or, each week) and mark when you ate and exercised as you planned, and when (and what happened) if you strayed off course. Also note what you ate instead of your planned meals, and if possible, the calories of the unplanned food. You can check the nutrition facts labels on the foods eaten, use the online USDA nutrient database for foods without labels (www.nal.usda.gov/fnic/foodcomp/search), look online for food at restaurants, or use *Restaurant Confidential* to guesstimate. Doing so will help you become familiar with the nutritional content of the foods you typically consume, will help you become more conscious of your daily choices, and will provide you a framework from which to adjust your intake in Step Four.

Step Four: Assess Your Progress

At the end of each week, step on the scale and record your weight in your weight loss log. You'll probably be tempted to step on the scale more than once a week, but don't do it! It's not possible for you to lose enough weight in one day for it to register on the scale. Daily increases and decreases will be due mostly to water lost or gained—not fat. Wait until your designated weighing day, and then weigh yourself at the same time in the morning, always on the same scale, and preferably in the buff. And the scale is not the only way to measure progress: take body measurements with a tape measure and assess the fit of your clothing, too. Assess your progress for the week. Have you reached your goals? Have you lost weight? If not, what can you change or do better in the next week? Review your food and exercise log and make adjustments as necessary.

Repeat steps two through four until your final weight loss goal weight is reached, then move to step five.

Step Five: Start Your Maintenance Plan

1. Once you reach your final weight loss goal, add 200 calories to your daily 1,650-calorie intake.
2. After a week, weigh yourself at your usual time, on your usual scale. If you have lost any weight, add another 200 calories to your daily calorie

intake, if you have gained any weight, drop your intake by around 100 calories.

3. Repeat until your weight has stabilized—that's the amount of calories you need each day for weight maintenance.

4. Continue to plan your meals one week at a time with your new weight-maintaining calorie level, and to weigh yourself once a week, at your usual time on your usual scale. This will help you stay on top of your weight and adjust your calorie intake and physical activity as need be.

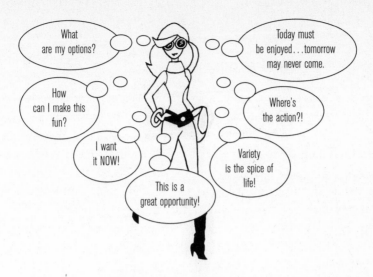

Inside a Diet Player's Head

CHAPTER 4

The Diet Players
ESFP, ISFP, ESTP, ISTP

In This Chapter...

THE DIET PLAYER PERSONALITY

- Pleasure Seeker
- Trouble Shooter
- Opportunistic
- Spontaneous
- Action Oriented
- Bold
- Competitive
- Adventurous

THE DIET PLAYER TROUBLE SPOTS

- Falling for Fads
- Eating in the Moment
- Over Indulging
- Getting Bored with Rules
  and Routine
- Wanting Immediate Results
- Getting Sidetracked from
  Health Goals

THE DIET PLAYER SOLUTION

- How to Win the Diet "Game!"
- The Diet Player Strategy

The Diet Player Personality

What's the easiest way to spot a Diet Player? Well, whether its recreation and dinner parties or work and a quick bite, a player personality likes to make sure she's having some fun along the way! Persuasive and open-minded, it's often the Players who are the performers, entertainers, and wheeler-dealers. The charismatic Player is often the center of attention, captivating her audience with stories, eliciting laughter and fostering camaraderie.

These likable risk-takers are motivated by adventure, excitement, and living in the moment. They are natural negotiators who seize opportunities, trust their impulses, and are skilled at deciding the best move to make in the moment. Whether these moves are on the stage (think Madonna), in the corporate suite (think Donald Trump), or on a sports field (think Michael Jordan), the Diet Players are highly resourceful and effective. If they "fail" to accomplish their goals they'll simply re-prioritize, bounce back and move on. Most Diet Players do not take lack of success personally. They'll just gather their energy, access the current situation and proceed from there.

> **Diet Players of Fame and Fortune:** Marilyn Monroe, Elizabeth Taylor, Amelia Earhart, Madonna, and Eva Peron all embody the characteristics of a Diet Player.

When someone with a Player personality embarks on a weight loss program, things sure can get interesting! Why? Well, true to their style, Diet Players like to eat, drink and be merry. This can certainly make it tricky to reach weight loss goals! As a Diet Player (I'm an ESFP) I can tell you first hand that this Diet Type wouldn't dream of being a "party pooper" by turning their noses up at tempting appetizers or by passing on an indulgent dessert at a social event. Quite the opposite; it's often the influencing Diet Player who will (loudly) encourage their friends, partner, or even the unsuspecting stranger next to them to join in on the pleasurable eating experience! Think about the last person who gushed at you, "Have you tasted the garlic shrimp? You simply must; they're just to DIE for!"

He or she was probably a Diet Player! Since they equate food with fun, asking them to turn down every indulgence, count calories, or stick to a rigid food plan will drain their delight and leave them feeling frustrated and caged.

> **Diet Players in the Movies and on TV:** Samantha in *Sex in the City*, Holly Golightly in *Breakfast at Tiffany's*, Satine in *Moulin Rouge*, and Scarlett in *Gone With the Wind*.

Let's get in the game with a Diet Player and take a look at how her player personality shapes her life, and how this effects her strategy to lose weight and eat healthy. After you read the summary of the Diet Player's basic internal "instructions," we'll look closely at what kinds of mistakes this personality makes when she aims to drop pounds.

As you read through the Diet Player's "stats," take the time to consider if, and how, each personality trait applies to you. If some of the qualities don't sync up with who you are as a Diet Player, don't panic! Your own unique combination of traits is just part of your individuality. Above all, your goal is simply to explore and *expose your personal weight loss challenges so you can learn how to use your personality strengths to have the energy to enjoy life to the fullest!*

DIET PLAYERS AT A GLANCE

Free spirit	Realistic
Process oriented	Uninhibited
Fun-loving	Practical
Good in a crisis	Enjoys the moment
Impulsive	Spontaneous
Needs freedom & space	Adaptable
Flexible	Seeks variety and change
Focus on immediacy	Most joyful

Source: Otto Kroeger Associates www.typetalk.com

Pleasure Seeker

❝ I live to eat! My social life revolves around delicious
   meals. **❞**
            —MICHELLE, A DIET PLAYER

If Diet Players had a motto, it would be something like, "Enjoy each
moment to the fullest." In tune with their senses of touch, smell, taste,
sight and sound, Diet Players are happiest when they have a chance to
indulge and experience life with abandon. As thrill seekers, they crave the
rush of adrenaline from an exciting encounter, be it a dangerous sky dive,
a risky relationship, or a decadent dessert. Diet Players don't spend a lot
of time questioning or second-guessing their instincts; they want to go for
it! Why miss out on the immediate pleasure of the caramel soufflé with
whipped cream? To stifle an urge or suppress a whim is to miss out on living, isn't it?

Diet Players are sometimes accused of "not being serious," but the truth
is they can be very serious about accomplishing their weight loss goals as
long as they can enjoy themselves in the process.

Trouble-Shooter

❝ I can make a meal out of just about anything. **❞**
            —DANIELLE, A DIET PLAYER

Diet Players naturally respond well in a crisis and can turn almost any
situation from a setback to a stepping stone. Incredibly resourceful in the
midst of chaos, they can think on their feet and come up with solutions at
the drop of a hat. Where others may hesitate and debate possible solutions,
Diet Players will take swift action. They'll take risks, reach out to whoever,
and do whatever it takes to quickly get the job done. You see this in movies
when a woman is forced to wear something drab and unattractive, before
she makes her entrance, she'll quickly rip her clothing, tie it, add some
extras and "voila" she has a hip, groovy outfit that steals the show!

If a Diet Player has *seriously* prioritized her health and fitness, she'll use
her go-get-'em energy to reach her goals, and she'll have a darn good time

doing it. Instead of sitting around thinking about what she could do to lose weight and get healthy, just like the Nike ads, she'll *"just do it."*

Opportunistic

> ❝ I tend to think wow that homemade peach-melba pie
> might not be here tomorrow... better have a piece now!❞
> —MELANIE, A DIET PLAYER

Diet Players don't like to miss out on anything. Whether it's a great sale on shoes, a primo parking spot, or free ice cream day—when a Diet Player spots an opportunity she wants to grab it before it disappears. One Diet Player described this as "opportunity eating." She said that any time an unexpected eating opportunity comes, like the chocolate cake someone brings as a surprise for a co-worker's birthday, unexpected free appetizers at happy hour, or the candy in the dish on the reception desk at the chiropractor's office, her philosophy is, "Hey, I might not get another chance, so I might as well indulge."

Diet Players are busy gals. They like to fit a whole lot into their lives. They would rather know they dove in and participated, taking a chance to turn a small opportunity into a great enterprise, than to sit back and watch life pass them by. This means if they catch wind of a new diet that is all the rage, they'll jump at the chance to try it.

Spontaneous

> ❝ I want to eat what I want, when I want it.❞
> —DANIELLE, A DIET PLAYER

Diet Players live in the moment—that is, right NOW, right this second! They like to be able to follow their impulses without worrying about the consequences. You can imagine that when it comes to food, a spontaneous Diet Player will most likely eat first, and think about her not-so-healthy choices later... if at all. Planning for a Player can take the fun out of things. They prefer instead to go with the situation, keeping their options open for whatever may come up in the moment. That's not to say the Diet Players aren't prepared. They are ready to participate or indulge in whatever attracts them in this instant and are primed to switch gears when necessary, so they can keep the object of their desires in their sights no matter what. And their "cravings" can change quickly; the circumstances call for it. Diet Players are usually "see food" eaters. . . if they see it and it looks inviting, they want to eat it!

Action Oriented

> **"** The high-impact work outs keep me interested. I need something like kickboxing or boot-camp fitness, something where I leave exhausted and sore. **"**
> —MELANIE, A DIET PLAYER

Action is the name of the game for Diet Players. They want to be a part of the action, not just watch it. Diet Players are notorious for doing many things at once—working many jobs, dating many men, or juggling multiple projects or activities. They are often the ultimate multi-taskers, talking on the phone, painting their nails, and checking their email. . . all at the same time.

Needless to say, a hectic schedule and a penchant for multi-tasking means Diet Players are often eating on the run. Navigating traffic while eating a muffin, grabbing a sandwich before hopping on a plane, or shopping for a new dress with a latte in hand, is no sweat for the Diet Player. At work, it is probably a Diet Player that is running errands, having a meeting, or reading a proposal while also eating her lunch.

Diet Players are most at ease when they are operating and interacting with the physical world. They are adept at using tools, gadgets, and instruments (even parts of their bodies) to manipulate and interact with their environments. Many great chefs are Diet Players. If you've ever watched the TV show Iron Chef, you've experienced a Diet Player's dream activity. It is a competition, against others as well as the clock. They work fast and use all kinds of gadgets, tools, pots, pans and appliances to create flavorful masterpieces. They choose from a variety of ingredients and have to think on their feet to create recipes from a special ingredient. And talk about the icing on the cake! They get to see, touch, taste, smell, and hear the food cooking. They work amidst chaos and commotion. . . lights, cameras and plenty of action. Then they describe their creations in great detail for the judges. Whew! What a rush!

Bold

> " If I really want to achieve something, I know I can do it as
> long as I have a true goal in mind. . . like finding a new job
> or running a marathon. "
> —MARIA, A DIET PLAYER

A trait of Diet Players that is admired by many is their confidence and determination. Appreciating expediency, Diet Players don't like to beat around the bush in conversations and interactions. They prefer to be direct and frank about their intentions, "Do you have a girlfriend? Do you want one?" Part of this is due to the fact that Diet Players are masters of the "fake it till you make it" philosophy." Another reason for her brazenness is that a Diet Player loves to get what she wants. One of the biggest motivators for a Diet Player to lose weight and adopt a healthy lifestyle is the ability to have the confidence she needs to be a winner in any situation. Some Diet Players are motivated because they want to look their best so they can impress and entice those around them

Pessimistic people and pessimistic dieters generally irritate the Diet Players. A Diet Player is not inclined to sit around and complain. How can they have a good time and reach their goals with a negative-Nelly bringing them down? It takes too much energy away from the more important things in life. . . like enjoying it! Diet Players also dislike awkwardness, cowardliness and indecisiveness. They don't like it in themselves and find it very unattractive in others.

Competitive

> " As long as I was competing with my best friend to lose
> weight by our class reunion, I was successful. "
> —MICHELLE, A DIET PLAYER

A contest, game, or competition will pique the interest of a Diet Player, who readily enjoys challenges and strives to be the best. Diet Players can put a lot of time and energy into practicing their technique and honing their skills, as long as they can keep a tangible goal in mind. Winning, and the adrenaline rush that goes with it, can be quite addicting to the "high-rolling" Diet Player—the higher the stakes, the bigger the rush! One saucy Diet Player shared that a girlfriend of hers bet she couldn't get past one day without drinking soda. The result? Our Diet Player sure showed her friend! She skipped sodas for an entire week. In fact, she kept going and hasn't had a soda since. Her motivation? Every time the Diet Player gets together with her friend she can brag about her feat.

Diet Players are drawn to others with a competitive edge—expecting they will make life more fun, interesting, or at least challenging—so they will do well with a competitor. Most Diet Player's would rather be playing a competitive sport (like tennis, softball, or golf) or engaging in a fun activity (like dance aerobics, snowboarding, or rollerblading), rather than running on a treadmill or pedaling on a stationary bike (yawn).

Adventurous

> **❝** I like to try new foods and experiment with my options. **❞**
> —JILL, A DIET PLAYER

If you are a Diet Player, you are well aware of your need for variety and change. Although some Types may find routine and schedules comforting because they know what to expect, Diet Players become restless and bored with structure. They need the flexibility, space and freedom to make choices, change options and create alternatives. When it comes to eating, Diet Players like to be a bit adventurous, they'll try hot and spicy on one day and sweet and creamy the next.

Diet Players like their activities to be diverse as well. Doing the same activity day in and day out is too mundane for a Diet Player. They are more likely to get their exercise in a variety of ways; they might go dancing one night, rock climbing the next day and skiing over the weekend. They aren't afraid to try the latest fad either. Whether it's the new "fat blocker" pill or the latest thingamajig exercise equipment from an infomercial, they welcome new tastes, activities and ideas. Eating the same foods and doing the same things over and over can feel like a jail sentence to a Diet Player. When it come to food and exercise, Diet Players need variety to keep them happy.

WHAT WORKS FOR DIET PLAYERS

Flexibility
Taking it one day at a time
Portion control
Competing with self and others
Short-term goals
Trying new things
Lots of activity

WHAT'S UP DOC?
Brandy's Story

❝ You've got to help me, Doc, I've gotta look *hot*—fast! **❞**

Some people are the life of the party…Brandy *is* the party! To many, Brandy can come across in one of two ways: either a breath of fresh air, or a tornado. I first met Brandy when she began her career as a pharmaceutical representative six years ago. Not one to follow rules, she would frequently finagle her way past my receptionist and into my office, where she would be waiting for me upon my return. Lively and funny, Brandy would surprise me with a new joke every time I saw her, and she often found the opportunity to give me a playful jab in the arm and exclaim, "Get outta here!"

Eventually I became Brandy's primary physician. As a Diet Player, she led a busy life and was always trying something new. With Brandy, it seemed, it was *always* something; from a broken ankle she got skiing, the back pain she developed after taking up kick-boxing, and a funny rash that she developed after a trip to Cancun.

But one day Brandy came in to see me for a different reason.

"Doc," she exclaimed, "my backside is HUGE!"

Her bluntness startled me.

"Excuse me?" I replied.

"And I've got a pooch!" she continued. "Can't you write me a prescription for an appetite suppressant or one of those fat blockers?"

Brandy had indeed been gaining weight over the years, and she was now about 30 pounds overweight. Being Brandy, it was typical that she expected the issue to be taken care of immediately.

"So Brandy, why is this coming up now? What motivated you to want to make this change?" I asked.

"I'm going to Palm Springs in a few months—and I want to look hot!"

I knew that the typical discussion about exercise, calorie restriction, and lifestyle modifications was going to fall on deaf ears. Brandy needed to do something *now*, get results *now*, and feel successful—*now*. Even a discussion about achieving a goal two months away (or even this weekend) was likely to be considered "long-range planning," a skill which did *not* fit Brandy's natural personality. We needed to tap into Brandy's innate ability to get things done *today*.

I took Brandy through a process called "mapping across." This entails pinpointing a previous accomplishment and applying the same approach used to attain success then, to another goal; in this case, the new goal was weight loss. We took the same skills she had used to successfully save for a down payment on a red convertible and applied them to saving calories so she could fit into her red swimsuit.

Brandy had effectively saved up for the car, *not* by crunching numbers and breaking down her budget, but by asking herself every day, "What can I do *today* to save money?" This attitude helped her resist spending. For example, when she saw a "gorgeous" pair of shoes and reached into her purse for her credit card, she immediately paused and thought of her bigger goal. "Really, how often am I going to wear those shoes?" she would ask herself, "If I buy them, I will have wasted the money I was going to put towards my car, and I will be further from my goal."

Brandy applied this same concept to eating junk food. Why waste calories? Instead of "using up" all her allotted calories for the day on a slice of cake, she would be more satisfied if she saved up those calories for more filling, healthful foods. She learned to stop and think "Wait a minute. Five minutes of a delicious dessert might be great, but it's going to move me further away from my weight loss goal!" Brandy's ultimate goal—to look great in her swimsuit—was clear to her, and she was free to make choices (for Diet Players, it is all about choices!). In summary, she was saving calories for a healthier food choice—just like she had made the choice to save money for her car by not buying shoes.

Several months passed before I saw Brandy again. She came rushing into the office and immediately and hit me with an enthusiastic high five, "I did it Doc!" she exclaimed, "I fit into that red swimsuit! And you know what?" she added with a big grin, "I looked *hot*!"

—Dr. Redard

The Diet Player Trouble Spots

Diet Players certainly have a lot going on, but the two most important things for them are having freedom, and being able to act—fast! Because Diet Players believe life should be lived to the fullest in the here and the now, they don't want any rules to hem them in. Once they find what they want to do, rather than discussing it, they just do it.

With those characteristics, the Diet Player can get off to a great start when it comes to weight loss. After all, she won't have any trouble getting herself to the gym because she is a woman of action. And she has such high energy the rest of the time that you would expect the pounds to just melt off of her.

The problems begin when a Diet Player starts to feel that she is being restricted or disciplined. Suddenly, she feels frustrated, and she gets off track. In the portion below, we will look at exactly how this happens. Then we will find ways for the Diet Player to predict her own weak tendencies—and beat them with her own strengths before they get the best of her.

Let's kick things off with a look at some of the Diet Player "trouble spots."

Just as you did in the previous section, take the time to consider how, and to what extent, each weakness may apply to you. And don't forget, you are a unique Diet Player among many other Players, so not every description will apply to you.

Falling for Fads

> ❝ I'll try any diet at least once! Why not? I've got nothing to
> lose... except maybe some weight!❞
> —LAURIE, A DIET PLAYER

While other Diet Types will talk (and talk and talk) about losing weight
and getting fit, if a Diet Player is serious about dropping pounds, she'll
skip the superfluous chatter and get right to it. A Player doesn't want to
debate diet theories, study various weight loss plans, or discuss the "what
ifs" of their health goals. They want to get started—NOW! However, in
their urgency to get the weight loss show on the road, they may not get all
the facts or they may make poor choices based on misinformation. This
can make attaining long-term effective results much, much more difficult
than need be.

Since Diet Players are so spontaneous, they can also go to the extreme
and make a quick decision like "I'm going to run a marathon in the spring!"
Although they start off with the energy and fervor of a runaway locomotive,
waiting and delays can be like a slow death to a Diet Player. She wants to see
"instant" results, and when she doesn't, she gets discouraged. Needless to
say, a Diet Player is susceptible to those quick fix (failure) fads that promise
you will lose "ten pounds in just ten days!"

Eating in the Moment

> ❝ I like the instant gratification of eating bad things.❞
> —MARIA, A DIET PLAYER

Diet Players with weight troubles tend to go from one indulgent food
moment to the next. If their lunch-time deli spot has a cheesy-steak sub
on special, they'll think, "why not?" If they see a tempting scone behind the
counter at their coffee spot, they'll give it a try and indulge without hesitat-
ing. And if their partner wants to order a deep-dish double-meat pizza for
dinner, they won't think twice about sharing in the fun.

When restrictions are put on a Diet Player that prevent her from grabbing the gusto from life, she begins to feel trapped. Naturally, weight loss

plans that ban entire food groups, require adherence to lots of rules, and allow no room for flexibility, will be unworkable for this Diet Type in the long run. Oftentimes, it doesn't take long for a Diet Player to find that a diet is too controlling for her. No matter how much enthusiasm she starts with, once she feels hemmed in, she will move on to more exciting and fulfilling ventures almost immediately—and leave her good diet intentions in the dust.

Over Indulging

> **"** I cannot stand to be deprived of the things I want, and that is what the word 'diet' means to me.**"**
> —NATALIE, A DIET PLAYER

It's easy to guess that a Diet Players bold tendencies and "seize the day" mindset can easily lead to overindulgence. Nearly every day is exciting and special to the action-driven Diet Player, and she often feels she has to act on her enthusiasm by celebrating—with a sweet treat or caloric concoction. In addition, on the days when the active Player is feeling more stressed than fabulous, she is also prone to consume too much just to help her cope. Occasional indulgence is not a big deal, (most of us are all too familiar with over-doing it on Thanksgiving or on other special occasions), but the constant cycle of spoiling herself with food is no good for the Diet Player, who will inevitably pack on the pounds faster than she would at an all-you-can-eat chocolate buffet.

Getting Bored with Rules and Routine

> **"** Diets take planning. You have to think about meals instead of just grabbing something quick.**"**
> —COLLEEN, A DIET PLAYER

It's not surprising that most Diet Players find it difficult and exasperating to follow traditional weight loss plans. Most (if not all) are based on lots of rules and regulations (yuck), and keeping track of points, carbs, or calories is this Diet Type's worst nightmare.

Also, because a Diet Player likes to have the freedom to do what she wants, when she wants, she can be resistant to making a weight loss commitment—and it's even harder for her to keep them. When a Diet Player makes a plan, they typically view it more as a flexible goal or suggestion, not something carved in stone. They may also set unrealistic goals, such as; "I will never eat sweets again!" Unfortunately, this means they often set themselves up for failure.

Wanting Immediate Results

> **"** If I start a diet and I don't see fast results, I'll just drop it and move onto something more satisfying.**"**
> —STEPHANIE, A DIET PLAYER

For a Diet Player, waiting for something to happen can feel like torture, especially when she's waiting for her new, svelte figure to emerge. A Diet Player wants results, and wants them yesterday. The danger is, unrealistic expectations about how long it will take to shed those extra pounds will do more harm to their waistline than not exercising or overindulging: the number one reason people ditch their "diet" is not because of a lack of time, knowledge or willpower, but because they get fed up when they don't lose the fat as fast as they thought they would. It's a shame because all that hard work goes down the drain, and starting again can feel really discouraging.

The desire for immediate results is part of the Diet Player's eagerness to make things happen. What she wants is action—now! Unfortunately, this also means that, when, for whatever reason, a Diet Player isn't able to be as physically active as she wants, she may eat just to have something to do—better than doing nothing! If they can't go out dancing, well, at least they can indulge in some chocolate. Cold outside... can't exercise? How about whipping up something delicious and having a feast instead! Stuck indoors doing boring paperwork? Spice it up with some yummy snacks!

Getting Sidetracked from Health Goals

" My work out plans often get de-railed when more exciting
prospects arise. "
—MELANIE, A DIET PLAYER

The Diet Players desire to indulge in the moment is so strong that sometimes their goals (like weight loss) get pushed aside in favor of what is
immediately stimulating (like chocolate or a dinner party).

Also, living life to the fullest in true Diet Player fashion means these
ladies often overextend themselves in several areas of their lives all at once.
Although Diet Players are equipped to strive with this kind of priority-
juggling, her health comes last when she's in a hurry. Exercise? Who has
the time when they have a business to run, a crises to solve, an opportunity
to grab? Eat right? How can they plan meals, they've got places to go and
people to see? This kind of willy-nilly approach to her health means our
Diet Player can form some very bad habits.

WHAT DOESN'T WORK FOR DIET PLAYERS

Scheduling
Long-range planning
Weight loss meetings
Rigid or complex food plans
Counting anything
Routine
Reviewing research or detailed diet data

WHAT'S UP DOC?

Crystal's Story: A Diet Player

" Ok, you have to tell me doc. Why can't I lose weight? I mean,
I've tried everything and it hasn't helped! What's up? "

Crystal's engaging personality draws you in with her enthusiasm and
larger than life adventures. She can talk about the most mundane things
and make them seemed so important and relevant at that moment. She

has honed these natural abilities to become a sought after speaker and corporate trainer.

With her optimism, self confidence and "can-do attitude," Crystal is fearless, yet she seems to get herself into one predicament after another. She accepts speaking engagements on topics that she's never presented, double books speaking engagements on the same day, or even schedules a talk in New York for the morning and half way across the country for that same evening. But her, shoot-from-the-hip style (and frequent adrenalin rushes!) get her through with accolades from her audiences. While her natural abilities allowed for success in many areas, other aspects of her life tended to get pushed aside, or simply denied—like her weight.

Crystal grew up thin. With no effort at all she stayed thin throughout her teens and early 20's. However, during her college years she started to put on weight. She wanted to be successful so she put her full effort into her schoolwork while working nights to pay her way; she found it quite natural to burn the candle at both ends. The only time she felt she could take a break and relax was to eat.

Soon she started to associate everyday activities with eating. For instance, she would come home after a long day and head straight to the refrigerator. In her unconscious mind, walking through the front door became associated with "EATING TIME!" She didn't even have to be hungry to eat, simply walking through the front door triggered her to want to eat. She could have just finished lunch, then walked outside to check the mail, walked back in the house and found herself unconsciously driven to look for something to eat. It became quite automatic. Same thing when she was driving. Simply hopping in the car triggered her hunger and she would forage for whatever was available—and it was usually bags of chips or cookies she had stashed somewhere.

It didn't help that her friends and relatives all gained weight along with her, so she remained the thinnest in her peer group. It was always easy to reason "I'm thinner than all my friends." It wasn't until a couple of her girlfriends went on a diet that it hit Crystal that she was heavy, she wasn't luscious, she was lumpy! It was time to do something about it.

As a New Year's resolution, Crystal really took weight loss seriously, counting calories and working out religiously. Before she knew it, she had arrived at her pre-college weight. Having reached her target she figured, "Whew, I can go back to my 'normal' way of eating now. The fight is over! I've won! No more deprivation!"

So what happened next? You guessed it, she gained the weight back. This pattern of dieting repeated itself over and over.

"I just don't get it," she exclaimed to me one day, "Why doesn't any diet work for me?"

"Hmm... it seems to me that every diet you went on 'worked.'"

"Yea, but when I went off it, I gained the weight back!"

"Ah, Crystal, right there you have the keys to the kingdom," I said, "The key to staying sexy and fit is to have a way of eating that is effortless, that is fun, that is automatic, and that you actually look forward to doing. That way you never have to 'go on' or 'go off' the diet. In fact, it's not even a diet, it's just the way you eat—it becomes your new 'normal.'"

"But it has always been such a struggle, I always have to work so hard at it!" she recounted.

"Always?" I questioned. "As a child you were thin and didn't ever think about it; your eating habits were just as natural and part of your life as walking and talking. It's just that *you've* added some habits over the years that *seem* to be a permanent part of you. Well, they aren't, and if you're willing we can unhook them right now."

I worked with her to break up these associations and hook them up to healthier behaviors such as stretching the moment she walks in the door and listening to her body cues for hunger instead.

Next we turned to the concept of "memory management"—thinking NOW how she will feel BEFORE she eats the food. Will she feel tired...bloated...regret for blowing her diet? She learned to let those awful feelings stop her BEFORE eating, freeing her to make choices that feel good now, AND later.

Crystal is now eating and exercising in her "normal" way. She lost the weight without a struggle or simply by using "willpower"—she just fit back into the real Crystal.

—Dr. Redard

The Diet Player Solution
Part One of Your Solution:
How to Win the Diet "Game!"

Now it's time to make the first move towards winning the diet "game" and developing your very own Diet Player Strategy. How? By starting with *you*, of course!

First, you will take a close look at who you are, how you live, and whether your life is fulfilling your Diet Player needs. It is this process that will help you overcome your trip-ups, or "Trouble Spots."

Then, with that knowledge in hand, you can move to your Diet Player Strategy: creating your own customized, foolproof diet solution. This includes specific weight loss and eating tips. In this way, you will work *with* yourself to attain your weight loss goals. That's because you can use your natural Diet Player skills to anticipate—and overcome—your weaknesses.

Remember, you know yourself better than anyone else. So how could there be anyone better to turn to for guidance? And, after all, you are the only one who can lead you to accomplishment.

Here's a reminder of those pesky weak spots for a Diet Player:

- Falling for Fads
- Eating in the Moment
- Over Indulging
- Getting Bored with Rules and Routine
- Wanting Immediate Results
- Getting Sidetracked from Health Goals

Let's take a closer look at some Player-friendly ideas for addressing key trouble spots by looking into your own life. Finding a way to get past your tough spots means developing important life skills that are in sync with who you are. As you read the below, decide if some (or all) of these things need to be addressed in your own life. Then, work through the advice, one solution at a time.

How does a Diet Player not fall for fads?

When your mind is made up that you want something, you want it NOW, but before you jump on the latest weight loss bandwagon at least know this—quick fix fads can quickly spell more pounds in the near future. It's time to get in the know, stay in the know, and take the action that will give you the most success.

〜 TAKE ACTION NOW

• Realize that quick-fix weight loss fads only offer short-term solutions. To lose weight in the long-term, you have to change your habits in the long-term.

• Ditch the fads and "get in the know" by checking out The Basics in Chapter 7. Bonus, once you're in the know, you'll not only be primed to lose the weight and keep it off, you'll also be able to impress all of your friends and family with your new-found knowledge and skills.

WHY FADS ARE FOOLISH

Rapid weight loss (more than two or three pounds a week), is mostly water loss, and losing water weight is not the same as losing the real weight enemy—i.e. fat. Not only will losing water weight leave you feeling dehydrated and drained, you'll regain the water weight just as fast as you lost it. Quick-fix diets also severely restrict calories and your unsuspecting body—who has no idea you're just trying to fit into your skinny jeans—will assume you are starving to death and automatically slow your metabolism, making it even more difficult for you to lose pounds. Even worse, when you start eating normally again your metabolism will remain sluggish to allow your "starving" body a chance to regain weight as fast as possible. In short, quick-fix fad diets only offer quick-fix solutions, and because they don't teach you how to change your habits in the *long-term*, they can't solve your problem in the *long-term*. As soon your old eating habits return, so does the weight.

GET IN THE KNOW

When it comes to weight loss and nutrition, even though *everyone* seems to be a real know it all, very few actually know the real deal. And, with all the confusing info out there in the wild, wild world of weight loss, it's easy to get turned around. The truth is, losing weight is not complicated. As long as you eat a (mostly) healthy diet and get moving, those extra pounds are gonna disappear. Don't worry—Chapter 7 provides you with all the facts you need to know. And, since you are a Diet Player who wants to get started *fast*, all the most important info is summarized in an easy-to-understand format for your convenience (see Know Three, page 93).

STAY IN THE KNOW

As a Diet Player, here's a quick way for you to keep up-to-speed on the latest health news when you are on the move: healthy living publications like *Self, Fitness Magazine, Good Housekeeping,* or *Cooking Light,* newsletters like the fantastic *Nutrition Action Healthletter* and e-newsletters, (like my favorite: The Hungry Girl), make it fun to stay on the cutting edge of nutrition. Plus, you don't have to read the material from cover to cover. Just by thumbing through, you'll pick up new exercise ideas, weight loss tips, healthy recipes, food news, as well as other tricks and tidbits. Why not indulge and get a subscription? It will save you cash and time because you don't have to remember to purchase one. Plus, it will give you something to look forward to each month!

How does a Diet Player keep from eating in the moment?

If you want to lose weight, something's gotta give, and following every urge into the land of calorie-laden foods is going to get you nowhere, fast. What to do? For your Diet Type, it's all about healthy options and strategy.

∼ TAKE ACTION NOW

Make everyday a chance to make a healthy change or build a healthy habit. Keep your goal in mind and make today count!

- Make today the day you clear out your cupboards and create a healthy home-base. Throw a "take or toss" party, where you invite neighbors or friends to take the foods you no longer want. Whatever they don't take, you will toss.
- Make today a chance to lighten your "out and about" calories. Pick up nutrition brochures from a few of your favorite restaurants, or check out the info on-line.
- Make today the day you increase your activity. Challenge yourself to find ten ways to incorporate more activity into your life today, whether it's aerobic, lifestyle, or an everyday activity.

GETTING IN THE GAME

Taking away all your favorite foods and forcing you to eat things you detest would be like a prison sentence to your Diet Type, but if you *don't* make some healthy changes and reduce your calories, the prison will be your own body. Since complicated plans won't work for the spur-of-the-moment Diet Player, you need a different type of strategy. Below, I have provided a great 1-2-3 game plan that is perfect for beating the Diet Player urge to eat at the drop of a hat. Because you are a Diet Player who likes options, we will have some more strategies for you when we outline your personal Diet Player solution (see page 92). But for now, implement these steps into your life to defeat those tempting, spur of the moment urges.

1-Your Home-Base Strategy

The best chance for your Diet Type to make smart, calorie-controlled choices is in your "home-base." Your "home base" includes where you live, but it also encompasses other places where you spend a lot of time, like your office, or place of work.

To make your home base work to your advantage, clear your space of the not-so-healthy foods you know will get you into trouble in the heat of the moment. Instead, stock up on healthy options you ENJOY and only keep the "junky" foods you can't live without around in portion-controlled quantities (the 100-calorie packages of cookies, chips, etc., make this easy to do.) Note that this is not a strategy you should employ only when you're trying to drop pounds—this behavior should become a life-long habit. Treat your home-base as your health sanctuary—considering the time you tend to spend "out and about," you're gonna need it.

Of course, the healthy options are limitless, and your favorites will be a matter of personal preference, but trust me here; you won't feel like you are sacrificing if you keep foods around you take pleasure in eating. If you're a gal who frequently has impromptu get-togethers, perhaps you'll stock up on hummus, crudités, whole grain pita chips, olives and nuts, so you *and* your guests can eat healthy and enjoy it, too. If you spend a lot of time in an office, this might mean keeping a bowl of fresh fruit on your desk, a stash of granola bars in your purse, and a stack of healthy frozen meals in the kitchen freezer. If you're a stay at home mom who enjoys cooking, you might stock up on interesting salad ingredients, bake crusty home-made whole grain bread, and make a trip to the fish market every few days. No matter what your lifestyle, at your home-base it's all about eating the *right* food in the moment.

HEATHER'S HEALTHY HOME-BASE

While it changes with the season and my mood, most of the time you can find the following items hanging out in my kitchen: whole grain pita, Sabre hummus, olives, mixed greens, baby spinach, arugula, edamame, jarred roasted peppers, grape tomatoes, eggs, smoked salmon, goat cheese, Parmesan cheese, pine nuts, almonds, walnuts, chicken-apple sausages, Amy's Lower in Sodium Soups, prosciutto, Barilla Whole Grain Pasta and Raos Pasta Sauce, Kashi Go Lean cereal, fat-free milk, Fage Total 0% Yogurt, Fiber-One Granola Bars, Pepperidge Farm Whole Wheat Cinnamon Swirl Bread, Land O' Lakes Light Butter with Canola Oil, honey-crisp apples, peaches, berries, tangerines, bananas, Skinny Cow Ice Cream Sandwiches, a stash of Lean Cuisine Spa Cuisines, and an assortment of 100-calorie portion-controlled treats and snacks.

2-Your Out and About Strategy

Once you've got your home-base strategy in place you need to think about what to do when you are out, and if you're like most social Diet Players, this is quite often. Again, educating yourself about food and calorie content will really help you, an "in the moment" gal, make better "in the moment" food choices. (One of my favorite expressions is: ignorance might be bliss, but it's also fattening! Want an example? The average order of eggplant parmigana with spaghetti has at least 1,000 calories and a Rueben sandwich has around 900. Considering you should only consume about 1,600 calories per day when you are trying to lose weight, those are some mighty big indulgences.)

Part of your out and about strategy is having enough knowledge to make painless calorie-saving swaps. Where do you get the facts? Scan the nutrition brochures or online nutrition info for some of your regular spots. Most "out and about" spots offer a selection of tasty good-for-you options—it's just up to you to make the choice to try them. This might mean trading in your Starbucks Venti whole-milk Café Mocha with whipped cream and a scone (940 calories) for a Grande Skinny Mocha and a biscotti (240 calories). Or maybe substituting your rib-eye steak with a loaded baked potato (1,230 calories), for a filet mignon with veggies (450 calories). It's important that you select food swaps that will leave you feeling satisfied because if you force yourself to eat foods you hate, you'll not only make yourself miserable in the short-term, you'll just go back to your old eating habits in the long-term.

There are times, however, when "just saying no" (or just saying "swap" for that matter) is not a realistic option. So what's a desperate-to-be-in-her-skinny-jeans Diet Player to do? Try these sensible (semi) solutions on for size:

Pair Down Portions—Portion control is a food lovers number one defense against weight gain. How does it work? You can eat what you love. . . just not a lot of it. Servings in most restaurants are gigantic, so no matter what you order, either split it with a friend, or for even more control, ask for half to be boxed up before it hits the table. Servers will most likely be polite about this. . . after all, good service is how they earn their living!

Mix it Up—If you can't stand going out for breakfast without having bacon, pair a few strips with a cup of oatmeal and fresh fruit. If a French bistro is not the same without the frites (fries), couple them with a rotisserie chicken (sans the skin) and mixed greens with dressing on the side. If you can't live without the crème brulee dessert, have grilled fish and vegetables as an entrée. You get the idea.

Try a Little, Leave a Little—Don't waste your calories on food you're not crazy about. At a cocktail party, buffet, or similar event, try small bites of the things that look good, but only finish what you really, really like. Don't munch away on foods that taste just so-so, simply because they're on your plate. Instead, save your calories for the things you thoroughly enjoy.

Implement Damage Control—If you have an indulgent meal or day, don't let it start a downward spiral. Your indulgences won't get a chance to stick to your hips if you choose low-calorie options for your next few meals and increase your level of activity for a few days to neutralize the impending damage. In fact, this strategy is a lot more reasonable than trying to avoid indulgences altogether. After all, what's a life without a little indulgence?

Pick Your Pleasures—From time to time it's good to give yourself a break and just eat, drink and be merry. Since you live life as it comes, you may not be able to plan these times, but as long as you don't feast more than once a week, it's A-OK to occasionally spoil yourself. It's a lot easier to be "better some of the time", than "perfect all of the time."

3- Your Activity Strategy
Exercise and activity means ladies with less-than-perfect diets can maintain closer-to-perfect physiques. That's because the more active you are, the more calories you burn—it's just that simple. The American College of Sports Medicine recommends 20-60 minutes of moderately intense (breaking a sweat) aerobic exercise 3-5 times a week. But here's a great trick: that 20-60 minutes doesn't need to happen all at once; it's just as beneficial to get it in smaller increments of 10-15 minutes at time. Choose smaller

portions of time to be active, 3-4 times per day (like taking a quick walk on a break instead of sitting in the lunchroom) and you'll have squeezed in a full work out without taking a big chunk of time out of your day. The more you work out and move, the more calories you burn—period. And if you include strength training (lifting weights) at least twice a week, you will build even more muscle and burn even more calories. Just like healthy eating, finding activities you actually enjoy is the key. Most Diet Players like to compete, like to be challenged, and like to be pushed to their limit, but the type of activity does not matter as much as making sure you get it in. *Aerobic* activities, like swimming, hiking, step aerobics, kick boxing, spinning, yoga, etc.—are all beneficial. But so are *lifestyle* activities, such as gardening, yard work, and washing your car. Same goes for *everyday* activities like taking the stairs and parking farther from the store entrance so you have further to walk. Take every opportunity to increase your daily activity, and you'll see a dramatic difference in your weight loss efforts—guaranteed.

Since life (like happy hour, and last minute dinner plans, business meetings, and get-togethers) can sometimes throw a wrench in your work out intentions, try keeping a bag of work out clothes, shoes, and gear in your office or car at all times. That way, you are ready to exercise whenever. (A worthy waistline investment is an extra pair of work out shoes—that way you can keep one pair in your office or car, and one in your house, so you are always ready to be ready!)

How does a Diet Player keep from over-indulging?

Too much of a good thing is, well, just too much! While we aren't talking about giving up eating, drinking, and being merry, it is necessary for you to get a handle on excessive over-eating. The following four little tricks will show you how.

~ TAKE ACTION NOW

- Keep yourself satisfied so you are better able to make healthy "in the moment" food and drink choices.
- Remember NOTHING tastes as good as skinny feels. The next time you are on the edge of an overindulgent pig out, put the brakes on by remembering *before*, how you are going to feel *after* overindulging, and by paying attention to your satiety senses. Your "Think Three" strategy on page 95 will help you jump-start your skills.
- So you don't feel deprived, find some yummy ways to make everyday a little indulgent.
- Optional Additional Reading: *French Women Don't Get Fat* by Mireille Guiliano

---

MANAGE YOUR HUNGER

One of the easiest ways to prevent overindulging is to keep yourself satisfied so your body doesn't panic and demand that you eat, *fast*. If you're frequently on the run, it's helpful to stock your purse, desk, car and etc., with an emergency stash of healthy "grab" foods. Fiber rich bars (like Fiber One and All Bran), and packages of nuts, whole grain crackers, and dried fruits are all good options. Also try putting a bowl of fruits with peels, like oranges and bananas, on a table near your front door, and always grab one on your way out. My personal arsenal of Chocolate Oats Fiber-One Bars has saved me from many a disastrous Krispy Kreme run-in.

Likewise, many Diet Players frequently make the fatal mistake of going hungry all day so they can "save" their calories for a social function later that same night. Trouble is, you're so ravenous by the time you get to the party, dinner, or event, that you end up eating a heck of a lot more than if you'd had a healthy breakfast and lunch earlier in the day. If you eat *before* an event you'll keep your appetite on an even keel and have much better control of your intake. Remember: To prevent overeating you simply need to eat.

TRY MEMORY MANAGEMENT

Imagine yourself overindulging. How do you feel after? Bloated, guilty, drained, disgusted, and, probably, FAT. Could you have received the same pleasure by eating a smaller amount? Eating way too much of anything is never a pleasant experience, and if you remember the negatives *before* you overindulge, and stop yourself *before* the damage is done, you'll save yourself a lot of agony. Typically, when people first try this trick, they "forget to remember" until after they've eaten too much, but once they "remember to remember" it gets easier and easier.

TAKE A BREAK
When you are plowing through a large portion of something delicious, it's easy to get carried away and eat way past fullness. Use your finely tuned Diet Player senses to pay attention to what your body's telling you. As soon as you start to feel even slightly full, or sense you are starting to eat just because it tastes good, put your fork, spoon, sandwich, or whatever you are eating, down and stop for a few minutes. Drink some water or make some small talk, and before you resume eating, check your hunger level and then decide if you really want to finish what's left on your plate.

INDULGE EVERYDAY
Although it sounds counter-intuitive, diet *without* denying yourself food pleasures! A Diet Player without her favorite foods will be miserable and give up fast. To avoid this, eat small amounts of the food you love and you'll satisfy your urge without doing the damage. Also, keep food on hand that will indulge your cravings without expanding your waistline, such as fat-free pudding cup or a mug of low-fat hot cocoa instead of a chocolate bar. I tame cookie and potato chip urges with those 100-calorie packs, and ice cream means a scoop or two of my favorite low-fat brand. A frequent after-dinner dessert is a bowl of fresh berries and a regular late-night snack is a handful of chocolate-covered almonds. Find your own ways to make everyday a little indulgent and you'll curb overeating by keeping the cookie (or chocolate, chips or whatever) monster at bay.

WHAT'S REALLY GOING ON HERE?
Sometimes, however, overindulgence has less to do with physical hunger and food cravings, and more to do with your state of mind. Are you in a deadbeat job, relationship, or living situation that is causing you stress? Are you overeating to fill a hole because you lack excitement in your life?

Instead of ignoring the unsatisfying parts of your life and overcompensating with food, take a good look inside, find what is stressing you out and do what you do best—take action! Kick it into high gear and make some changes so you can get back into a positive state of being. You have the freedom and the power to create your own fulfilling, healthy life—so go for it!

How does a Diet Player keep from getting bored?

If you find typical diet plans boring and frustrating, get ready to break all the rules and make things fun!

> **～ TAKE ACTION NOW**
>
> • Come up with a list of things to keep your healthy lifestyle interesting and fun. Post the list where you're sure to see it each day, and add, change and update the list on an ongoing basis. The sky's the limit on your healthy ideas and choices!
> • Be conscious of when eating has become a response to something other than hunger. Check out your "Think Three" strategy on page 95 for extra help.
> • Jumpstart your weight loss with a friendly competition.

BREAK THE RULES

Ah, diet rules. The lists of weight loss do's, don'ts, must's, must not's, should and shouldn'ts are endless. Here are just a few: Never eat before bedtime. Eliminate bread, pasta, or anything that even resembles a carbohydrate. Record every morsel of food that passes your lips. Only eat grapefruits. Only drink green tea. If you're like most Diet Players who have tried to follow the diet rules, you've probably started out by saying to yourself, "this time I will buckle down and lose this weight once and for all." And with all the fervor of Mario Andretti on race day you throw yourself at the mercy of *the rules*. What happens next? It might go like this: You refuse all forbidden foods, you turn down social events to avoid tempting situations, you force yourself to run on a treadmill two hours a day, you eat mashed yeast and drink herbal shakes—in short, you follow the rules. But, after a few painful days (or for you real die-hards, a few painful weeks or months), you reach your breaking point and toss aside that good-for nothing, unworkable, stu-pid, preposterous, *living-torture* diet and go back to living a life—thank you very much!

While *reasonable* rules can be essential tools for some people, (hint: "only eat grapefruits" is *not* reasonable) for a Diet Player they're akin to a death sentence. Do yourself a favor and forget "the rules!" More important than following a list of do's and don'ts or sticking to a routine is finding ways to keep yourself continuously excited and engaged in your healthy lifestyle. Living a healthy life can be every bit as flexible and enjoyable as living an unhealthy one. It's all about choices and balance. If you have eggs Benedict for breakfast, have a light lunch and dinner. Tired of spinning class? Try biking or dance aerobics. Sick of going to the gym? Rent a work out video or go for a run outside. Dying for a cookie? Have one or two instead of ten. Don't feel like working out today? Skip it, go for a brisk walk in a new neighborhood, and hit the gym tomorrow.

Keep it Interesting

Changing your lifestyle can actually be a lot of fun for your Diet Type. Making a change means trying different things, experimenting with new activities, foods, and restaurants, and adopting a new, healthy point of view. While other Diet Types will naturally resist and even fear change, Diet Players will embrace what's new and different. For Players, "new" equals fun. More good news: there are a million ways to keep your healthier life interesting, challenging, new and fun! Try new food products, new grocery stores, and new farmers markets. Try new cooking gadgets, new cookbooks, and new recipes. Go rock climbing, start a garden, or go for a hike. Enlist your friends to train for a half marathon, start a healthy cooking club, or take a cooking class. Hire a trainer, buy cute work out duds, or join a cool gym. Sign up for a golf league, a tennis team, or a soccer group.

Try making a list of activities, classes, or whatever sounds like fun to you, and post it where you're sure to see it on a daily basis. Add to this list whenever you think of something else you might want to "give a whirl." Try things out, discard what you don't like, and embrace what you love. The possibilities and choices are endless; in fact, I've had a running list posted to my fridge for the last five years. Some of the things on my list I never seem to get to (oh well), others I end up doing again and again, and lots of things I'm involved in are not even on the list. The point of the list is to help you find, remember, and explore interesting, healthy activities, because once you're engaged in an active lifestyle that you enjoy, the pounds will drop off naturally. And once you taste the sweetness of success, you won't want to go back to the bitter struggle.

HEATHER'S HEALTHY FUN LIST

* *Take an Asian cooking class—check L'Academie de Cuisine schedule*
* *~~Plant herbs on garden rooftop~~ Buy herb cookbook—ask Tamara for recommendations*
* *Find new hiking trails in Blue Ridge mountains*
* *~~Try Rock Creek restaurant (owned by an RD)~~ Love it! Don't forget to order the shrimp appetizer next time!*
* *~~Take Pilates class~~ YUCK!*
* *Sign up for spinning classes with Mia*
* *Find health spa for weekend get-away with Cyndi*
* *Go to Linden Winery for apple picking in early Fall*
* *Register for Natural Food Products show in Baltimore in Aug.*

MAKE IT A COMPETITION

Jump start your healthy way of life and your weight loss by setting up a (a-hem) *friendly* competition with a friend, coworker, or your spouse. Make a wager and let the contest begin! Bet a co-worker $20 that you can avoid the breakfast room pastries longer. Wager $50 to see if you and a friend can both go two weeks without eating "junk" food. Bet your spouse $100 that you can work out more times in a month than they can. Set whatever challenge will drive you to implement good behaviors, and then use the momentum you gain and the strategies you learn from the competition to keep going. The next thing you know, you'll have created a healthy example for yourself.

UNHOOK THE FOOD CONNECTION

Not only do Diet Players get bored with routine, you also tend to eat when you are bored. Notice whether food has become connected to an activity even when you are not hungry, such as going to the movies and eating popcorn, snacking on candy while watching TV, or going out for drinks and ordering appetizers. Do you even notice you are eating? Or has the food become a mindless habit? Again, use your finely tuned Diet Player senses to pay attention to your hunger. Notice when you are eating due to hunger (good) or due to boredom, social reasons, or simply because there is food available (bad). Sometimes just noticing our habitual responses can help break our automatic actions and reactions.

How does a Diet Player build patience?

As much as Diet Players love variety, they can also become scattered and distracted when they have too many choices or there are too many demands on their time. To prevent anxiousness and a feeling of being overwhelmed, a Diet Player needs to make sure that life's variety is grounded in sound prioritizing.

⌁ TAKE ACTION NOW

- Focus on the short-term, realistic health and weight loss goals.
- Think about the one (or even two or three things) you can do today that will help you reach your goals. Keep your goal in mind and make today count!

FOCUS ON SMALL REALISTIC GOALS

While I'm sure you have an ultimate goal in mind—going down a dress size, reaching a desired weight, fitting into a favorite pair of jeans—to help you reach your goal "faster," try setting small, achievable goals. One way is to aim to lose 5 percent of your start weight. If your starting weight is 180 pounds, you'll want to aim for a loss of 5 percent of 180—or 9 pounds. Expect an average loss of about two pounds per week. Therefore, you can assume a REASONABLE time frame of about 4 or 5 weeks to lose 9 pounds. After you reach your first goal, set a new goal using the same formula. Keep going, one small goal at a time, until you reach (and you WILL reach) your ultimate goal.

FOCUS ON SUCCESS

Imagine success, expect it, and work for it. Diet Players have a tendency to leave decisions to the last minute so they can choose whatever they "feel like" in the moment. Those who are most successful at maintaining a healthy weight, imagine themselves making a healthy food choice, (no matter what options are presented), expect this behavior from themselves, and imagine succeeding ahead of time. They may not know the specifics, but when the time comes, they follow through—and succeed! Always keep your eye on the prize.

FOCUS ON MORE THAN THE SCALE

The scale alone is not the best way to measure your weight loss progress. Why? It only tells you total body weight, and doesn't specify inches lost or muscle gained. A tape measure and the fit of your clothes will give you a more complete picture of your progress. Also keep in mind that weekly (not daily) weigh-ins provides a better gauge of where you're at in the pounds department. Just be sure to weigh yourself at the same time (preferably in the morning), on the same day of the week, using the same scale. And for best results, weigh yourself in the buff.

FOCUS ON TODAY

Daily goals like: "take spinning class this afternoon," "sign up for a cooking class this morning," "eat five servings of fruits and veggies today" are practical and helpful. Setting and achieving daily health and weight loss goals helps you stay focused on today, and each goal you put into practice will result in healthy habits that in turn, will move you closer to your larger goal. Post daily helpful reminders like a sticky note on your computer "drink more water!" dashboard "yoga class at 6 today!" or your door "grab a piece of fruit!" Remember that every day, every hour, and every second is a chance to turn it all around. You will get to your final weight loss goal when you get there—but you need today to help you get there.

How does a Diet Player stay on track?

It's time to build your own personal recipe for success. We all have had the experience of achieving goals in one or more areas of our lives and in order to accomplish those goals we had to do certain things, believe certain things, and focus on certain things. When combined together, your beliefs, actions and attitudes that you adopted to achieve your goal is your personal success formula or "success recipe" for achieving ANY goal, including weight loss.

~ TAKE ACTION NOW

- Brainstorm past achieved goals and see if you can apply the same process to weight loss.
- Find your success recipe, decide to make your health and your weight loss a priority, and then make it happen, one day at a time.

BUILD YOUR SUCCESS RECIPE

Think of a time in your life when you accomplished a desired goal such as saving money for a down payment on a car (see Brandy's story), getting a job you wanted, or learning a new skill. Once you have your previously accomplished goal in mind, think about how you were able to achieve that goal and see if the same "recipe" for success could be applied to your weight loss efforts. Take Dr. Redard's Diet Player client Dana. Dana came to see Dr. Redard because she was desperate to drop 20 pounds before her wedding. Chatting with Dana he found out that a few years back she had taken up snowboarding. He asked her to tell him exactly how she had learned to snowboard—to kind of outline the process. Dana thought for a few seconds and said, "Sure, it was easy! First I took a couple snowboarding lessons so I could figure out what the heck I was doing—although it turned out I was a natural (wink)—and next I started going snowboarding with my friends who were already boarding pros. That way I could pick up their techniques and learn all sorts of neat tips and tricks while boarding with them. I also saved up so I could buy lift tickets at a local mountain. I was in college and waitressing at night, so every time I came home from work I would immediately put half of my tips in my snowboarding jar on the hall table, right next to my snowboard. Anyway, with more money in hand to spend on lift tickets I would go to the mountain and practice, practice, practice. Now it's been 3 years since I started and I'm a darn good snowboarder, if I do say so myself!"

He asked Dana if she could use this same method to help her lose weight—and she did. She figured out what "the heck she was doing" by reading some info he gave her on weight loss and by joining a gym and having a trainer to show her the ropes. She started to chat with women on a wedding planning blog about the things they were doing to slim down before the big day, and based on another bride's recommendation she signed up for a boot camp program—she loved it and starting going four times a week. She also started to check out the calories on food labels and online at some of her favorite eateries and she found lower calorie choices she really liked. She cut her portions in half whenever she ate out and she kept a list of low-cal "go to" meals on her fridge. Every time she lost a pound she would put $20 into a weight loss jar she kept on the kitchen table. When she had a "bad" day (and she had plenty of bad days) she would shake if off, spend a little more time working out, and remind herself of her larger goal. Four months later Dana had lost the 20 pounds and she spent her $400 weight loss savings on some new clothes for her new smaller size. To help Dana maintain her weight, each week she stays at her desired weight she puts five dollars in her weight loss jar and every six months she uses the money on whatever she wants—a weekend spa trip and a new snowboard are some of her recent splurges.

Of course, your own weight loss "recipe" will depend on your own unique experiences and accomplished goals. And keep in mind if one recipe is not as useful as you expected, toss it aside and mix up another. As a pragmatic Diet Player you have the ability to tackle problems, clear hurdles, and knock down barriers—doing whatever it takes to reach a successful outcome.

Part Two of Your Solution: The Diet Player Strategy

Now that you've anticipated all the ways you might block yourself from success, nothing can hold you back! Let's develop your perfect weight loss strategy. It's as easy as 1, 2, 3!

Know Three

The Basics in Chapter 7 provide the low-down on weight loss and nutrition in a fun an easy-to-understand format that you will help you in your day-to-day life. Spend a little time reviewing the Basics (c'mon, I know you've got 20 minutes to spare!) and keep the following overview in mind.

The Only Three Diet Tricks You Need to Know…

EAT MORE OF…

1

Colorful Fruits and Veggies. Produce is not only nutrient dense—meaning, it packs a large number of nutrients (e.g., vitamins, minerals, antioxidants, etc.) into a small number of calories—it's also high in fiber and water, so it fills you up. The more variety, the better.

Whole Grains. They're more filling, more healthful, and better tasting than refined grains because they have not had their fiber-and-nutrient-rich bran and germ removed by processing. Eat whole grain versions of bread, rice, cereal, pasta, and flour as often as possible.

Lean Protein. Lean choices like beef (filet mignon, sirloin and London broil) pork (pork loin, tenderloin, center loin and ham), poultry (boneless skinless chicken, turkey cutlets, and ground turkey and chicken), deli meats (turkey, roast beef and ham) and all types of fish and shellfish are packed with protein, not calories.

Low-Fat Dairy. The best way to take advantage of dairy's good-for-you benefits (protein, calcium, and other essential nutrients) without any of the bad-for-you fat (saturated fat and cholesterol) and excess calories, is to choose more low-fat or fat-free dairy products, more often.

Beans. Low in fat and calories, but chock full of filling fiber and good-for-you phytonutrients, vitamins, minerals, and protein—as food goes, beans are near perfect.

Good Fats. For satiety, taste and good health, pick foods rich in mono-unsaturated or polyunsaturated fat: avocados, oils like olive, canola, corn, sunflower and soy, nuts, and Omega-3 fats derived from fish and flax.

EAT LESS OF…

Sugary Foods. Sweetened cereals, cookies, candy, muffins, cakes, pies and other sugary foods not only wreck havoc on your blood sugar, but they're also loaded with nutrient-poor calories. Same goes for refined grains like white bread and white pasta.

Fried Foods. French fries, fried chicken, chips, doughnuts and all other deep-fried foods are packed with calories, not nutrients. And the oil used to fry foods in most restaurants and fast food joints is loaded with artery-clogging trans fat.

Fake Foods. Processed foods and "junk" full of partially hydrogenated fats, chemicals, and preservatives are just not as nutritious as whole real foods.

Full-Fat Dairy. Cheesy and creamy usually means fatty and full of calories. Cut back on full-fat butter, cheese, cream, yogurt, whole-milk, and ice cream. For lots of flavor and less calories, try using strong cheeses like blue, feta, Parmesan, and feta in smaller amounts.

WATCH YOUR DRINKS

Liquid calories are hiding in your coffee drinks, your cocktails, your sodas, your fruit smoothies, and even in your "hydrating" sports drinks. Take a look:

12 ounce glass of juice with breakfast: 170 calories

16 ounce café latte with whole milk for snack: 260 calories

16 ounce sweetened iced tea with lunch: 120 calories

12 ounce fruit smoothie for afternoon snack: 300 calories

8 ounce glass of red wine with dinner: 170 calories

Total Hidden Calories: 1,200 calories

That's a HUGE dent in your daily 1,600 calorie quota you need to uphold in order to drop pounds! One of the easiest ways to shave calories is to change what you drink, and leave the calories to food. Stick with lots of water, or no-cal or low-cal drinks like my favorites, Hint and Honest Tea

tea, coffee and lattes with skim milk and Splenda, and an occasional *small* glass of juice, and cut back or cut out of everything else.

And don't forget about alcoholic drinks. Alcohol has been shown to stimulate the appetite and is often paired with high calorie, sugary mixers and is accompanied by calorie-laden bar snacks. That means it's easy to take in a lot of calories with just a couple of drinks and a few handfuls of munchies. Alcohol is always best consumed in moderation, and women who choose a cocktail should stick to no more than one per day. Choices like light beer and a small glass of wine are better lower calorie options than liquor drinks that can be brimming in calories. (One margarita can easily contain as many (or more) calories as an entire meal.)

Think Three

Losing weight is about more than just eating right and exercising, it's about THINKING thin.

You might be surprised to learn that you make over 200 food decisions in a single day. Don't believe it? Consider how many choices you make just ordering your morning cup of Joe at Starbucks. First you select your drink (latte) then you pick the type of milk (skim) then you choose the size (Grande) then you decide if you want to throw in a doughnut, pastry, or muffin to go with your coffee (no thanks) and then finally you decide if you want a flavored syrup, Splenda, raw sugar, white sugar, or Sweet n Low in your drink (sugar-free caramel syrup please). That's a TON of decisions right there!

Diet Players who manage to lose weight and keep it off, and those who have never struggled with their weight, make *conscious* food choices. They have a very good idea of just how much they eat and drink and if they overeat on occasion, they'll compensate later by eating less or exercising more to make up for it. Players who struggle with their weight, on the other hand, deliberately try not to think about how much they eat. Their food choices are based purely on what sounds good in the moment.

Just as it is possible to delude yourself about your food choices, it is also possible to train yourself to pay attention. Before you make a food decision, take a second helping, put a bite in your mouth, or put a drink to your lips, ask yourself the following three questions, and in a matter of just seconds you'll arm yourself with the consciousness needed to make better choices in the moment.

WHY AM I ABOUT TO EAT THIS?
Diet Players often eat or drink simply because they are bored or just because the food is there and it looks good. Remind yourself that the best reason to eat is because of hunger, and then make your choice with your weight loss goal in mind.

WHAT ELSE CAN I CHOOSE?
Diet Players like options, so before you make a food decision, consider all your selections. Also think about what else you had to eat that day and how your choice will fit into your over all day, and then make your choice with your weight loss goal in mind.

HOW WILL I FEEL ABOUT THIS CHOICE LATER?
Diet Players have a tendency to forget about their weight loss goals when they are in the food moment. Consider how your choice will impact your very near future, and think about how you will feel after eating too much (bloated, guilty, FAT), and then make your choice with your weight loss goal in mind.

You'll be amazed how your choices change with just a tiny bit of consciousness. Even when you make indulgent choices you'll be primed to take the action needed after (eating less or working out more or both) to minimize the damage. The more you practice "Thinking Three", the easier it gets, and eventually it will click into place and become second nature, much like riding a bike or driving a car.

Pick Three

Eat more of the good stuff, eat less of the bad stuff, and get moving, and you will lose weight—it's not rocket science. But if it's been a while (or ever) since you've watched portions, selected healthy picks or made conscious food decisions, it helps to have some flexible guidance to help you get back in the weight loss game.

It's difficult to determine precisely how many calories you eat, or precisely how many calories you burn, so don't get too concerned with exact numbers. Instead, simply "Pick Three" breakfasts, lunches, dinners, snacks, and Craving Tamers (Craving Tamers help you to keep all your indulgent foods in your life by simply slimming down the portions) that you can "go to" whenever hunger strikes. Post your choices on the fridge, carry a copy in your purse, or put one in your desk. Fill your fridge, cabinets (and your car, purse, office and etc.) with the ingredients and foods you need to prepare you Pick Three choices, and when hunger strikes, just choose whatever sounds good at the time.

You can use the Pick Three Easy choices below, or you can mix-and-match your Pick Three choices from the more structured meals in Chapter 8 (Some people do better on a lower-carb diet—see page 207—so there are picks for carb-lovers and protein-lovers alike). When you tire of your Pick Three choices, you just toss them out and Pick Three more. It's easy and the choices are endless! You can have your picks at any time and in any combo. Want to have breakfast for lunch, and lunch with your snack? Go ahead. Feel like having your Craving Tamer at breakfast? Or want to save your daily Craving Tamers for a larger indulgence one day in the week? No problem. When and where you want to eat your meals is totally up to you. Pair your picks with increased activity (page 223) and decreased "out and about" calories (page 81) and you'll drop pounds, feel satisfied, and reach your goals in no time flat.

THREE EASY BREAKFASTS (ABOUT 400 CALORIES)

Egg-y	Cereal-y	Smooth-y
2 eggs cooked any way, 1 slice whole grain bread, 1 cup fruit of choice (or 1 piece medium whole fruit), 1 tbsp. nuts, and 1 cup fat free milk	*1 cup high-fiber cereal with 1 cup fruit of choice and 1 tbsp. nuts topped with 1 cup fat free milk*	*1 cup lowfat vanilla yogurt mixed with 1 cup frozen berries and 1 tbsp. honey. Serve with 1 slice whole grain toast spread with 1 tsp. butter*

THREE EASY LUNCHES (ABOUT 450 CALORIES)

Salad-y	Sandwich-y	Soup-y
3 cups mixed greens tossed with 2 cups chopped vegetables of choice, 1 oz. crumbled cheese of choice, and 2 oz. lean meat, poultry or fish of choice (or ¾ cup beans). Drizzle with 2 tsp. oil and 2 tbsp. vinegar. Serve with 1 cup fruit of choice (or 1 piece medium whole fruit)	*1 slice whole grain bread topped with 3 oz. lean meat, poultry, or fish of choice, 1 oz. reduced fat cheese, lettuce, sliced tomato, and onion. Serve with 1½ cups cooked vegetables of choice drizzled with ½ tbsp. olive oil*	*1 cup bean or vegetable soup of choice, 1 slice whole grain bread, ¼ cup hummus, ½ cup sliced vegetables of choice, and 1 cup fruit of choice (or 1 piece medium whole fruit)*

THREE EASY DINNERS (ABOUT 550 CALORIES)

Pasta-y	Meat-y	Veggi-y
1 cup cooked whole grain pasta tossed with 2 cups cooked vegetables of choice, ¾ cup pasta sauce, and 2 tbsp. Parmesan cheese. Serve with 2 cups mixed greens tossed with 1 tbsp. oil and a splash of vinegar	6 oz. lean meat, poultry or fish of choice, ½ cup cooked whole wheat couscous or brown rice, and 3 cups cooked vegetables of choice tossed with 2 tsp. butter or trans-free margarine	1 veggie burger topped with 1 oz. reduced fat cheese and 1 cup sliced raw vegetables served on a whole wheat roll. Serve with 2 cups mixed greens tossed with 2 tbsp. light dressing of choice and 1 cup fruit of choice (or 1 piece medium whole fruit)

THREE EASY SNACKS (ABOUT 150 CALORIES)

Fruit-y	Cheese-y	Coffee-y
1 cup fruit of choice (or 1 piece medium whole fruit) with 1 oz. reduced-fat cheese	4 whole grain crackers topped with 1 oz. reduced-fat cheese	Medium (16 oz.) café latte with skim milk with a shot of sugar-free flavored syrup

THREE EASY CRAVING TAMERS (ABOUT 100 CALORIES)

Sweet-y	Salt-y	Ice Cream-y
2 miniature chocolate bars or 1 fat-free pudding cup	1 oz. potato or tortilla chips	½ cup light or low-fat ice cream

Note: for lots more meal choices see Chapter 8 on page 239.

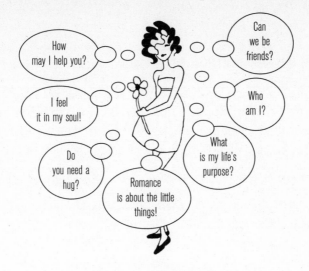

Inside a Diet Feeler's Head

CHAPTER 5

The Diet Feelers
ENFJ, INFJ, ENFP, INFP

In This Chapter...

THE DIET FEELER PERSONALITY

- Relationship Centered
- Guided by Emotion
- Peace Keeper
- Altruistic
- Craves Connection
- Searches for Self
- Sensitive
- Embraces Possibilities

THE DIET FEELER TROUBLE SPOTS

- Ignoring Your Own Needs
- Emotional Eating
- Denial of Your Health Issues
- Social Food Struggles
- Trouble Staying Self-Motivated
- Low Self-Esteem
- Waiting for "Tomorrow"

THE DIET FEELER SOLUTION

- How to Move Past Your Roadblocks
- The Diet Feeler Journey

The Diet Feeler Personality

Overall, Diet Feelers are idealistic, optimistic, and strive to make the world a better place. When treated with kindness, they are among the easiest people in the world to get along with—they truly are "True Blue" friends. They exude warmth and compassion, and their adaptable nature makes them a pleasure to be around. The Diet Feelers want to discover who they are, and how they can become the best they can be. Yet they're not only concerned about becoming better people themselves; they also encourage others to develop their own authentic individuality.

Diet Feelers of Fame and Fortune: Princess Diana, Audrey Hepburn, Jane Fonda, Eleanor Roosevelt and Oprah Winfrey, all embody the characteristics of a Diet Feeler.

Diet Feelers are generous, supportive, and caring individuals who enjoy being needed and like to please; often, they try to be everything to everyone. They are at their best when they are ardently involved in their interests, freely able to express themselves, and feel they are in alignment with their personal values and spiritual ideals. If they're not careful, however, these super-feelers can get over-involved and over-whelmed, leaving no time or energy for themselves. And in the world of weight loss and food this can lead to big (pun-intended) trouble. They often have a tug a war within themselves—how do they take care of others and yet at the same time take care of themselves?

Good nutrition and exercise are important for *anyone* who wants to take care of their health and lose weight, but for the Diet Feeler especially it's critically important to examine the "why" behind their habits. For the Diet Feeler, eating is a way to connect and socialize with others, and sharing a meal expresses intimacy, creates camaraderie, and brings friends closer. Food is a reward, a gift, and a pleasure to be enjoyed and appreciated. Food can also be seductive, a friend that a Diet Feeler can count on, and a comfort they can turn to. Combine this with the Diet Feelers desire to please, which makes it extra hard to say "no" to food prepared by loved ones or to turn down an invitation to dine with a friend, parent or a spouse, and you can begin to understand some of the reasons this Diet Type might find herself embroiled in a weight loss battle.

Diet Feelers in the Movies and on TV: Carrie from *Sex in the City,* Viola in *Shakespeare in Love,* and Karen in *Out of Africa.*

Below, you'll find a summary of the Diet Feelers key qualities. Take a look at how the Diet Feelers way of viewing the world shapes her life and how this affects her weight loss goals. Then, we'll examine some of the common Diet Feeler diet and health weak spots. Keep in mind that you are unique, and we all have all four Diet Types within us to some degree, so all of the following traits may not apply to you. Remember your goal is to start a personal journey of self exploration and to expose and identify your personal weight loss barriers, needs, and desires, and understand how to use your distinctive personality strengths for lasting healthy weight success.

DIET FEELERS AT A GLANCE

Seductive	Vivid imagination
Interpersonal skills	Mysterious
Supportive of others	Hypersensitive to conflict
Sympathetic	Autonomy
Relationships	Needs encouragement and
Interaction	recognition
Cooperation	Integrity
"Becoming"	Giving strokes freely

Source: Otto Kroeger Associates www.typetalk.com

Relationship Centered

> " My friend made a casserole for the company potluck.
> Nobody was eating it, and by the look on her face I could
> tell she was disappointed. I didn't want her to feel bad so
> I dished up a couple of big scoops... It tasted awful, but I
> ate it anyway and felt good about it."
>   —LIZ, A DIET FEELER

People are incredibly important to Diet Feelers, and Diet Feelers are supportive, accepting and thoughtful friends, parents, spouses, and co-workers. When making decisions (even small ones) their main concern is on keeping their relationships intact and others happy. They are energized and motivated when they are able to help and satisfy others, and it brings Diet Feelers joy to put a smile on someone's face. Diet Feelers often are the ones who eat a piece of cake because they don't want to hurt someone's feelings, or a second or third helping of pie, lasagna or whatever, just to please someone else. You get the idea.

You can count on a Diet Feeler to be there for you, especially in times of need. It's usually the caretaking Feeler who will bring chicken soup to a sick friend or share a pint of ice cream with a heartbroken sister. That's because the Diet Feelers, much more than any other Diet Type, connect food with comfort, and equate their loved ones' comfort with their own personal happiness.

Guided by Emotion

> " Food 'cures' or 'anesthetizes' pain. I eat when I'm unhappy.
> I eat when I'm happy. Eating is always a pleasure. Hunger
> is not usually a main reason to eat."
>   —LAUREN, A DIET FEELER

Enthusiastic, effervescent and full of life, Diet Feelers are drawn to the passion and drama of life. They admire the beauty, as well as the difficulty of existence, and strive to find meaning in life's moments. The act of fully experiencing a range of emotions, from elation to melancholy, and sharing their feelings with others makes these women feel most alive. Whether she is experiencing misery or bliss, the array of possible human emotions can be a trigger to eat, and every emotion seems to have a food connected to it. Furthermore, if there is no-one present for her to share her feelings with, she can celebrate or commiserate, with food as her companion.

Peace Keeper

> " Every time I get in a bad relationship that involves conflict,
> I turn to food to deal with the stress, and I gain weight. "
> —MIA, A DIET FEELER

Diet Feelers seek harmony and agreement. They function best in an environment that feels peaceful and safe for everyone. Confrontation, conflict, and lack of cooperation can be tough for a Diet Feeler who likes to maintain harmonious relationships and may make great sacrifices to do so. Flexible and accommodating, when it comes to choosing a place to eat, a Diet Feeler may say, "Well, where do you want to eat? You choose. Any where you want is fine with me." For a Diet Feeler, they've already made what to them is the most important decision—to go out to eat with you; the place or food is not nearly as important to them as your time together.

When conflict doesn't involve them, Diet Feelers may try different approaches to restore harmony for others. We've all heard the saying "Food soothes the savage beast," right? Well, Diet Feelers might bring a big batch of brownies to work to lighten the mood (they may consume a few themselves on the drive in). If that doesn't work they'll try to mediate a discussion, but again, if their help is rejected or worse—they are met with hostility—they can shut down and drop out of participation. And this type of rejection could lead to (you guessed it!) eating comfort foods. For a Feeler conflict equals stress, and if they're not careful, stress might also equal more brownies, doughnuts, pizza or candy.

Altruistic

> ❝ I go all day without eating and then eat one huge meal at
> night. I'm just too busy running around from one thing to
> another. ❞
> —SARAH, A DIET FEELER

Helpful, generous, and compassionate, Diet Feelers have a charitable, humanitarian spirit. They can be found volunteering their time serving food at homeless shelters, joining "walk-a-thons" to benefit those with illness or disease, and sending money overseas to aid starving children. Whether it is keeping their own home and family life intact, or helping world causes, they feel such a drive and a need to contribute that many Diet Feelers are willing to give of their time at their own expense. This means they often neglect their physical health and emotional well-being.

Craves Connection

> ❝ I have a gym buddy that I work out with each morning. As
> long as she's there, I'm there. She keeps me motivated. ❞
> —BROOKE, A DIET FEELER

Because the world of a Diet Feeler revolves around their relationships, from immediate family to friends, their community and even the world, they experience an incredible amount of stress if they have no one to share their lives with. A Diet Feeler is in bliss when she's in a loving relationship and she easily shows affection. Nothing spells romance to a Diet Feeler like an intimate candle lit dinner! From a romantic meal, to a family gathering, to a party with friends, some of the most bonding times for Diet Feelers are when they are eating with others.

Having friends with a positive attitude towards healthy eating is one of the biggest indicators for success in reaching her weight management and health goals. If her friendships are strong and she is esteemed by them, she may even take on the role of mentor to help rally them around to healthy habits.

Searches for Self

❝ When I am on my path and following my 'purpose', my eating just falls into place naturally. ❞
—AMBER, A DIET FEELER

"Who am I?" is a familiar question for Diet Feelers who seek to find purpose and meaning in their lives and actions. This introspective nature compels them to dig deep in search of their unique identity. Although Diet Feelers yearn to fit in, get along with others, and support friends, they have a conflicting, tugging desire to be extraordinary or one-of-a kind in some way. When it comes to food, this means they often pride themselves in having a special recipe that is exclusively their own, and features their own special touch. As for dieting, this urge to be unique may compel a Diet Feeler to decide that she—unlike everyone else—has an undeniable "inability" to lose weight, and that she is cursed to be "forever" overweight. Furthermore, since a Diet Feeler sees the *whole* person in herself and others, she is apt to think, "People should just like me the way I am. I am not my body."

Sensitive

❝ I spent hours making a nutritious meal for my family. They ate unenthusiastically. They never said they didn't like it, but I could tell they really hated it. ❞
—SARAH, A DIET FEELER

Diet Feelers have an intuitive nature. They seem to instinctively know when someone is trying to communicate something beyond the words they are saying. For instance, if someone says they are "fine," a Diet Feeler will pick up on the tone or inflection of the person's voice and use that to ascertain whether or not he or she is truly "fine." Although this talent comes in handy for understanding the needs of others, it also means that Diet Feelers pick up on "vibes" about themselves from those around them whether the other person has an opinion or not. Then, whatever the Diet Feeler perceives, she will take personally. For a Diet Feeler, who does her best to accept others, the sense that they are not being treated kindly, or others are being critical or judgmental, hurts—a lot. Add food to the equation and a Diet Feeler is very likely to eat for comfort when she feels injured or emotionally wounded.

Embraces Possibility

    " My friend really wanted me to try this avant-garde new
    diet. I didn't lose any weight, but it was fun exploring
    new avenues for growth and understanding other
    approaches.**"**
        —MARY, A DIET FEELER

Diet Feelers have a strong, hopeful optimism, and live in their vision of what a brighter tomorrow *could* be. As far as dieting goes, Diet Feelers have trouble getting off to a good start because their head is so often "in the future." Because they believe in the inherent goodness of mankind, they'll give people a second, third and even a fourth chance, noticing improvement where others may have given up, often because they perceive improvements in the other person's behavior that most would not notice.

    When it comes to health, the Diet Feelers are likely to seek alternative methods for well-being, such as intuitive readings, energy healings, or chakra tune-ups. They are also drawn to spiritual practices such as Tai Chi, meditation and yoga.

WHAT WORKS FOR DIET FEELERS

Buddy system and daily encouragement
Non-food rewards
Sharing feelings, issues and ideas
Weight loss support groups
Creative solutions and journaling
Focusing on the future

WHAT'S UP DOC?
Diane's Story: A Diet Feeler

" I'm overweight and I can't stand it anymore! **"**

Diane, a Diet Feeler in her mid 40's was about 50 pounds overweight—but you would never guess that it bothered her at all. Diane always has a smile on her face and a bounce in her step, and everyone who meets her is drawn to her warm, attentive demeanor. A careful listener, Diane makes eye contact, and nods empathetically, making anyone feel that she understands his or her point of view immediately. In her conversations, which often centered on her husband and her two teenage sons, she pauses and encourages others to share a personal story or two. Despite a demanding job in Human Resources, a typical day often finds her taking a trip to the bank on a break to make a deposit for her brother, dropping a friend off at a dentist appointment during lunch, and checking the mail and watering the plants for a neighbor on vacation after work. *All* before arriving home to make dinner for her family.

Diane had been coming in for regular check-ups since her back injury 10 years ago. Our appointments usually began with a cheerful conversation and ended with a warm hug. But one day, our visit was different.

Diane smiled and chatted cheerfully as always, but there was something absent in her eyes. Sitting down next to her, I asked her gently and sincerely, "Diane, what's going on?"

There was a moment of silence as her eyes began to well up. I could see her struggling to produce an upbeat response. Finally, she gave up, and her words burst out as forcefully as her tears.

"I'm fat and I hate it!" she sobbed.

Warm and loving Diet Feelers like Diane try to keep a positive attitude, even when they may be feeling down. They have a tendency to *do...and do...and do* for others, often at the expense of their own desires. It feels good to give, but when someone sacrifices too much of themselves, it doesn't feel so good any more. The tears that Diane now shed were not just for today...she had been holding them back for years.

Between sobs, she related, "You know I injured my back almost 10 years ago. Before that, I weighed exactly the same as at my high school prom. After the accident, I started gaining weight and I felt sorry for myself. So what did I do? I ate more! I started eating tons of "comfort foods" like ice cream, chocolate and baked goods. Trying to be helpful, my husband often brought "treats" home to help cheer me up. On one level it was sweet of him to care, but inside I was screaming, 'Stop it! Don't you love me?'"

Although Diane's back had gotten better, her self-esteem had gotten worse. She hated looking in the mirror, and would often criticize herself, saying things like, "I'm getting so FAT—It's disgusting! Look how fat I am!"

Her back injury had set a cycle in motion; feel horrible—eat to feel better—gain weight—feel horrible—eat more—gain weight—feel horrible...

Today was going to be a turning point in her life.

I worked with Diane on changing her belief that the needs of others are more important than her own. We worked on strengthening her ability to say NO and personalized some affirming self statements to shift her derogatory self talk. I also helped Diane become aware that, rather than *taking care* of others to help them, she could help them by stepping aside and allowing them to act on their own and develop capacities for helping themselves.

She reinforced the lessons learned during our office visits by reading several self-development books.

In a healthier frame of mind about herself, her goals, and her needs, and with friends and family in place to support her, we tackled Diane's diet and exercise routine. She changed her diet slowly, one week at a time, with the help of a support group and a neighborhood power-walking club. Although it was difficult at first to "find the time," Diane noticed that the exercise really cleared her head and gave her time to concentrate and focus better. The better she felt about herself, the more weight she lost. A new cycle was established: feel good—eat healthy—feel terrific—look terrific—feel good!

The last time I saw Diane she was not only back to a healthy weight; she was also back to a healthy frame of mind.

—Dr. Redard

The Diet Feeler Trouble Spots

Although each Diet Feeler is unique and although she has many aspects to her personality, a Diet Feeler places the most value on relationships. Before they make a decision or take action, they consider the people involved and how they might be affected. They also spend a great amount of their energy searching for their true identity and purpose in life. This means that if a Diet Feeler realizes the positive impact a healthier lifestyle will have on her life and the lives of those important to her, she is sure to succeed! But, a Diet Feeler gets off track when she focuses too much on other people and not enough on herself. Let's take a look at some of her weight loss weak spots.

Just as you did in the previous section, as you read through the following, take the time to consider how, and to what extent, each weakness may apply to you. And don't forget, although you are a Diet Feeler, you are also uniquely you, so you may not be able to fully relate to every example. And that's just fine.

After you review these Diet Feeler slip-ups, you'll gain a deeper understanding about yourself. You will be ready to make the positive changes that will set you free from your weight challenges, and it will be second nature to blossom into a healthier, happier you!

Ignoring Your Own Needs

> " I have 3 kids, a husband, 2 dogs and a cat—they all need
> me and get cranky if they don't get fed. I am trying to find
> a way to balance my health needs with those of the ones
> around me...and it's not easy."
> —NICOLE, A DIET FEELER

Although her sensitive nature means the Diet Feeler is most likely very well in touch with her own desire to lose weight, her tendency to take on the burdens of others means there is little time left for her own needs. Diet Feelers can get overloaded, drained, and tired when they are spread so thin; because they are often so focused on others, they neglect or minimize the importance of their own well-being. For example, if a Diet Feeler's own desire to make nutritious meals clashes with the preferences of her mate or children, she tends to push her own needs aside and cook what her partner or her family wants. Also, it can be difficult for a Diet Feeler to ask directly for what she wants, since she often assumes (or hopes) that, because she is intuitive, other people will pick up on her hints, too.

Diet Feelers want to please EVERYONE so saying "no" can be stressful. And, although the reality of time and money means "doing it all" is impossible, because Diet Feelers believe in possibility, they will always try to find a way. Even worse, when they are unable to help they can suffer tremendous guilt and remorse, convinced that somehow, some way, they could have done more.

Emotional Eating

“ I try to listen to my body, to what it wants, but my emotions just get in the way. If I'm having a down day or angry at someone, food makes it better—even if I'm not hungry. It's like my head says *don't eat that*, but my heart says *go for it!*”
—MARY, A DIET FEELER

While many Diet Types struggle with emotional eating, for the deep-feeling Diet Feelers it can be particularly troublesome. When they are bored, the chips might come out; stressed, maybe it's fast food; sad: macaroni and cheese; in love: chocolate; heartbreak: chocolate AND ice cream; and conflict: anything close at hand.

One of the things that can drive a Diet Feeler to consume large amounts of "comfort foods" is rejection, isolation, or feeling left out. Diet Feelers like to be a part, to be connected with others. When they feel invisible or are perceived to be treated like an outsider, the pain can stab deeply. If their efforts to reconcile or be accepted fail, instead of causing further conflict or creating negative feelings in others, the Diet Feelers may secretly soothe their wounded spirit with food. That's because they have a tendency to suppress their intense emotions around a painful situation with the comforts connected with eating. Some Diet Feelers are also good at "going numb" and can easily lose track of their nutritional intentions as they fade out somewhere between seeing a cookie and eating it. They may consume three or four cookies before they even realize it.

Denial of Your Health Issues

> **“** It's very easy for me to put things off and ignore them when the negativity and problems before me are too much. I over-compensate and pretend my weight problem doesn't exist. **”**
> —LIZ, A DIET FEELER

As positive thinkers, it is the Diet Feelers who are most likely to pretend their weight problem does not exist. When they buy new clothes and discover they are a larger size, they'll tell themselves they are just cutting the clothes bigger these days. When a friend or co-worker mentions their weight gain, they might shrug it off and blame it on an ill-fitting outfit. Denial is often employed by a Feeler to avoid dealing with the negative energy they fear surrounds their weight issue. And this type of denial is exactly what will keep them from starting down a healthier path. Unfortunately, sometimes it's not until tragedy strikes, possibly the diagnosis of type two diabetes or a heart attack—that Diet Feelers are able to see themselves in a more realistic light.

Social Food Struggles

> **“** In my family our lives were centered around food. We connected through food. **”**
> —BROOKE, A DIET FEELER

The desire for food starts with a trigger of some kind. Besides the most obvious biological trigger (i.e. hunger) there are visual triggers (like seeing a juicy burger on a commercial), sensory triggers (like smelling freshly baked bread), emotional triggers (like feeling sad or lonely) and social triggers (wanting to eat what everyone else is eating). For Diet Feelers, social triggers are very powerful. For example, if everyone else is diving into a pumpkin pie at the Thanksgiving dinner table, even if the Diet Feeler is not hungry, and even if she doesn't *really* like pumpkin pie, she'll have a piece so she can connect and celebrate with the group.

Naturally, friends are an incredibly important aspect in the life of a Diet Feeler, and if her social circle cringes at nutritious food choices and the thought of exercise, her road to weight loss might be a bumpy one. If she feels she will be shunned or rejected by eating differently, she'll likely take the path of least resistance, even if it means ditching her own health goals.

Trouble Staying Self-Motivated

> **"** I used to exercise with a buddy each morning, and I was very faithful with going, but now she has moved away and I have not found anyone else who is interested in exercising with me. I do not have the motivation to do it alone. **"**
> —AMBER, A DIET FEELER

Diet Feelers, who are usually not motivated to lose weight solely by a desire to please themselves, but rather for a greater cause or for someone they love, often have trouble with self motivation.

They tend to think that guarding their own health is a small, selfish goal, and they may pay little attention to it because they are focusing on bigger causes. How could they even *think* about exercising when there is an important PTA meeting they have to attend? Their commitment to helping out means they will catch a quick bite on the way to the animal shelter to volunteer on "adopt-a-pet" day, or skip a meal altogether to help set up for the bereavement support group—only to binge later because they neglected their appetite. Doing so much for everyone else (and for the world!) can leave little time for a Diet Feeler's own needs. The worst part is, even when they realize they are on a downward spiral, they can feel selfish taking care of themselves. Sadly, feeling torn this way can plunge them into a funk or even depression.

Low Self-Esteem

> **"** My boyfriend criticized me on a daily basis. My self-esteem
> was so low I turned to food to numb out. **"**
> —SARAH, A DIET FEELER

Diet Feelers strive to express their true essence, and they become extremely stressed when they feel it is unsafe to do so. They are incredibly sensitive to hostility, tension "in the air," and aggression directed towards them, and even the slightest disapproval can be taken personally. This, along with their own feeling of not being "good enough," can take its toll and lead to low self-esteem. And, when they are vulnerable in this way, criticism about their weight can make them feel even worse about themselves.

Often, a Diet Feeler will make another person, group or cause her passion, doing everything within her power to make sure that others' lives are happy and fulfilled. Seeing others happy brings a Diet Feeler joy—until she realizes that she has lost herself in the other person or cause and has no true identity of her own. When a Diet Feeler is not following her true path and feeling passionate about her life, she may eat to satisfy her true desires and to fill the void.

Waiting for "Tomorrow"

> **"** I know that I am not at my 'perfect' weight, but I will deal
> with it tomorrow. **"**
> —LILY, A DIET FEELER

While all Diet Types can be guilty of waiting for tomorrow ("I'll start exercising tomorrow, I'll eat more fruit and vegetables tomorrow, I'll stop skipping meals tomorrow, I'll drink more water tomorrow"), the forward-thinking Diet Feelers are particularly susceptible to this diet downfall. Some Diet Feelers will bargain with themselves in their head thinking, "Oh come on, one bite of a cookie won't hurt" (They can believe that because they are truly *living in the possibility* that they can stop after just one bite). Ten cookies later, they resolve to start dieting again... tomorrow. Usually, that "tomorrow" never comes, and five days, five months, or five years later, a Diet Feeler will suddenly realize what's happened, and regret that she didn't start to make healthy lifestyle changes a long time ago.

Inspired by imagination and intrigued by what is possible, Diet Feelers get bummed out when nay-sayers point out all the reasons an idea will not work. Diet Feelers prefer to focus on what could be, and they can become frustrated when others roll their eyes at their "unrealistic dreams." They are also easily convinced by new diet pills, herbs and Weight loss "discoveries" and often fall prey to latest "miracle" diet.

WHAT DOESN'T WORK FOR DIET FEELERS

One size fits all approach
Competition
Criticism
Reviewing detailed diet data
Concentrating on just the body
Negativity

WHAT'S UP DOC?

Loretta's Story: A Diet Feeler

"Nothing works for me! I have tried everything!**"**

Loretta's bracelets jingled as she threw her arms in the air, sighing in defeat. Her flowing skirt and brightly colored scarves moved with her body as she acted out her agony with flair of an actress in a death scene.

"I've been cursed with the affliction of fat my whole life!" she said," It has stood in my way of finding my true love, discovering my true calling, and of expressing my true self. And now I am 50! Life is passing me by!"

A creative writing instructor at a local college, Loretta is also a writing coach and has authored several books herself, mostly romance novels. She also meditates, cooks, takes Tai Chi lessons, and enjoys free form dance classes. Creative, insightful, and intuitive, Loretta is a Diet Feeler, seeking to understand life and be understood. Her driving question is "Who am I?" and, even in the way she dresses, Loretta strives to be unique and different.

Indeed, every meeting with Loretta is different than the one before and I never quite know what to expect. One visit she is dressed in a business suit, the next she's in a mini-skirt and go-go boots. Just like her ever-changing wardrobe, Loretta's emotions change often as well. At times she is excited about life, love, and possibilities, and other times she is miserably depressed. One thing is for sure—the visit will be emotionally intense.

Like many Diet Feelers, Loretta has been on a journey to find her true self for years. This quest is particularly challenging because of her unique past. During a traumatic childhood, Loretta developed the tendency to "zone out" as a way of protecting herself from pain. On top of that, Loretta developed the tendency to turn to food for comfort. No matter what she was feeling, food was always there to soothe her. For Loretta, food didn't ask questions or judge, and it could always be relied on.

As an adult, Loretta has the same tendency to zone out and escape her feelings through comfort food. If her boss yells at her, instead of confronting him, she will run to the break room for doughnuts. If a date doesn't call her back, she will finish off a pint of Ben and Jerry's. After an argument with a friend, candy is her refuge.

On top of these destructive habits, Loretta had been deriving a sense of her "uniqueness" from her failure to manage her weight. Like many Diet Feelers, she found herself caught in a pattern of getting an emotional rush from sorrow, and using everyday crises as a way to manufacture dramatic situations. It was time for Loretta to know herself better and create a new identity around her *successes,* not her failures.

We began by exploring more resourceful ways for Loretta feel alive besides her emotional roller coaster. I recommended a tape series based on Neuro-linguistic Programing by Dr. Tad James called "*The Secret of Creating Your Future.*" By doing the processes explained on the tapes, Loretta was able to clear past negative emotions such as sadness, guilt and fear. Then I had Loretta track her emotional eating habits and learn to replace food with fulfilling and constructive activities, such as mediating and talking with friends. Soon, Loretta was losing pounds.

Along with the weight, she was also losing a lifetime of discontent. Now, as Loretta puts it, "instead of constantly struggling to break through, I feel like a flower "in full bloom." She still has her emotional intensity; along with the radiance, color and confidence to express her "true self" in healthy ways. If you met her, you would see it too.

—Dr. Redard

The Diet Feeler Solution:

Part One of Your Solution:
How to Move Past Your Roadblocks

Now that you've seen the strengths and trouble spots for your personality type, let's take a look at how you can beat those rough spots. Let's take a look at your roadblocks again...

- Ignoring Your Own Needs
- Emotional Eating
- Denial of Your Health Issues
- Social Food Struggles
- Trouble Staying Self-Motivated
- Low Self-Esteem
- Waiting for "Tomorrow"

As you read the following solutions and ideas, let your mind begin to imagine applying the concepts in your life. At the end of this section, in Phase 2 of your Diet Feeler Journey, you'll be asked to take an inventory of the challenges that affect you the most and you'll be prompted to come back to do the suggested activities, and to also digest and use all of the resources in this book that you will need for ultimate success. So, for now, just enjoy discovering the many facets of you, and prepare for your weight loss metamorphosis.

How does a Diet Feeler stop ignoring her own needs?

If you consider your own health a small, selfish goal, think about this. *The most selfish act you can commit is not taking care of yourself.* That's right. If you want to use your talents to make a difference in the lives of others, you must first take care of yourself. And it's not just your physical health that's important, it's also your mental and emotional health. Taking care of yourself supplies you with the strength and the perspective you need to keep going and to keep giving. If you're thinking, "I'm too busy" or "I don't have time," you're just making excuses. Taking care of yourself is a choice, so instead of ignoring your health, choose to love yourself enough to make the time for your health needs.

~ GET IN TOUCH

- Examine your personal health priorities and possible barriers. Try on potential solutions and apply the ones that work best for you.
- Practice setting boundaries: See Make Friends with "No" activity page 153.
- Learn to listen to your body's needs.
- Optional additional reading: *The Aladdin Factor* by Jack Canfield, *The Best Life Diet* by Bob Greene, and *When I Say No, I Feel Guilty* by Manuel J. Smith.

FIND YOUR HEALTHY PATH

Not surprisingly, a Feeler's path to a healthy lifestyle is an emotional journey involving personal growth and self discovery. Oprah (she displays all the characteristics of an über-Diet Feeler) says it best in the introduction of Bob Greene's, her inspirational health mentor's book, *The Best Life Diet.* *"You cannot ever live the life of your dreams without coming face to face with the truth. Every unwanted pound creates another layer of lies. It's only when you peel back those layers that you will be set free: Free to work out, free to eat responsibly, free to live the life you want and deserve to live. Tell the truth and you'll learn to eat to satisfy your physical hunger and stop burying your hopes and dreams beneath layers of fat."*

Start by examining your current obligations, overall priorities, emotional needs, and the big picture of your life, and consider (*really* consider) how often you overlook your own needs to please others. Begin to think about your personal health priorities, needs, wants, and desires and the potential barriers that could keep you from achieving your goals. Also think about the choices and the changes you may need to make in your life in order to give yourself the time to accomplish your personal health goals. Be honest, and mull over your possible barriers before you come up with some possible solutions you can use in the future to deal with these roadblocks. Diet Feelers are particularly skilled at creating unique ways of solving challenges, so do what you do best and come up with some creative, personalized solutions. Finally, consider how employing these changes would improve your life and the lives of those around you.

So if you want to start preparing nutritious meals for yourself and for your family (priority), but you also don't want to upset your loved ones who might not be so gung-ho about jumping on the health band wagon (barrier), a solution might be to get a hold of some tasty *and* healthy recipes (see Chapter 8, page 239) and introducing these new recipes slowly until you build a group of meals that are pleasing to all parties involved. The healthy, pleasing meals can be gradually phased in, while the not-so-healthy meals are slowly weeded out. Bonus: finding good-for-you meals the entire family enjoys is not only good for your health, but also the health of your loved ones!

Of course your list of health priorities and possible barriers and solutions are as individual and unique as you are. Keep in mind a journey has many different paths and routes, so if you find one possible solution does not pan out the way you hoped, there are plenty of others to explore and try.

MAKE FRIENDS WITH NO

Another important skill to help you on your healthier path is learning how to say NO. Recognize that saying NO is not a selfish act, but rather a necessary part of your personal growth. Saying NO not only helps you avoid second and third helpings and deal with "food pushers," but also helps you prioritize the things that are important to you (like your health!) and provides you with the time you need to concentrate on your goals. The way to get healthy and lose weight is to take the time and energy to focus on your goals; and the best way to help anyone else, is to help yourself first. (See Make Friends with "No" activity page 153.)

LISTEN TO YOUR BODY

What is your body trying to tell you? That's right, it's communicating with you all the time and it lets you know when you are tired, hot, cold, thirsty and hungry. Plowing through your day ignoring your body's signals, and getting by on caffeine or quick fixes sets you up for binge-eating later in day when you'll be starving, tired, and drained. In this weakened state it's especially difficult (almost impossible) to resist the tempting not-so-healthy foods that will be screaming your name.

The solution, of course, is to slow down, sit down, and enjoy a balanced, satisfying meal or snack. Even if you take just ten minutes to re-fuel with nutrient-rich options, you'll find you'll have a lot more pep in your step. In today's fast paced world where a sit-down meal is not always an option, it is also a good idea to always have a back-up plan. Try stashing some healthy options where you can get to them when need be. I carry Fiber One Bars and an orange in my purse at all times. My mom keeps a can of Ensure in her car and in her golf bag.

How does a Diet Feeler stop emotional eating?

As you've learned, for the Diet Feelers, food is often more than just fuel—it's also a friend, an escape and a comfort. It's time to realize that the comfort found in food is only temporary and does nothing to resolve the underlying issues, or to heal your hurt feelings. In fact, the overeating can actually cause even more bad feelings (such as shame and guilt), which will create a vicious cycle. Here's how to stop the madness:

~ GET IN TOUCH

- Track your personal food triggers and substitute emotional eating with healthier activities.
- Clear your environment of the foods you reach for in response to your feelings.
- Practice being mindful when you eat and eat only until you are satisfied, not stuffed.
- Optional additional reading: *Breaking Free From Emotional Eating* by Geenen Roth.

BREAK THE EMOTIONAL EATING CYCLE

1- Track your triggers: If you're an emotional eater, situations or circumstances can "trigger" uncomfortable emotions, thus leading you to overeat in order to avoid those feelings. Do you eat when you're angry, sad, lonely, bored, guilt-ridden, frustrated, or stressed? Whatever your triggers, an important part of breaking your emotional eating patterns is identifying what's pushing you to turn to food.

Start by keeping track of the times you eat, but are not actually hungry. Record the times you responded to a situation or circumstance by overeating or making an unwise food choice, and then answer the following questions:

Q: What occurred directly before you ate?

Q: What were you feeling at the time?

Q: What did you actually consume?

Q: Afterwards what were your thoughts, feelings and self talk?

See how well you can accurately capture your feelings and reasons for eating (besides physical hunger) for at least an entire week (see example chart below). If it's been awhile since you've eaten because of actual physical hunger, use the hunger scale below to help you out.

THE HUNGER SCALE
0- Famished/Starving
1- Very Hungry
2- Slightly Hungry
3- Satisfied
4- Very Full
5- Stuffed!

EXAMPLE:

Time	Level on Hunger Scale	What occurred before I ate (Trigger)	What I was feeling at the time (Emotions)	What I actually ate	How I felt after eating
6:25 am	*3*	*Thoughts of work presentation this morning.*	*Nervous Scared Anxious*	*Handful of chips. 3 cookies. 1 scoop of ice cream.*	*Fat. Guilty. Angry at myself.*
7:40 pm	*3*	*Unpleasant telephone conversation with mother.*	*Anger Guilt Fear*	*Practically half a box of cereal. 2 fun size candy bars.*	*Fat. Disappointed. Shameful.*

Important: approach this as a learning tool and try not to beat yourself up or feel guilty or angry with yourself as you track your triggers.

2- Uncover your cravings: Once you've recorded your triggers and emotions, it's time to review what you have written and dig a little deeper to gain some insight. At this stage, many Diet Feelers realize that their "appetite" was for something other than food. Instead of meeting their true needs (like a break, a fresh activity, or a hug), they tried to satisfy their emotional "craving" by eating.

Begin by taking a look at the list of emotions that triggered you to eat and brainstorm at least five *other* feelings or circumstances that are connected to that emotion. (Yes! *Five!*) That's because the first ones on the list are usually the most obvious and general, such as "boredom" or "stress." But as you continue to dig a little deeper, your list will become more specific and personal. Then, for each of the additional feelings or circumstances you uncover, come up with a positive or affirming outcome or outlook you can apply to each. Doing this will help you to "blow the cover" on the emotion because once you break the bad feeling down, you will see that it is actually manageable, and not something to be feared. This creates less stress surrounding that emotion, and fewer reasons for you to turn to food for comfort.

A great way to do this is to create a flow chart for each of your emotional triggers (see page 122 for an example).

Be aware that your feelings might be a sign that something is awry in your life, and that you may have to make some life changes. Or, your feelings may just be a reaction to normal levels of stress. Either way, digging deeper and dealing with how you feel will help to snap you out of your emotional daze before you blindly reach for the chips, ice cream, or other comfort foods.

3- Pioneer a new path: Next, take a look at your list of emotional triggers and mark the one you would like to address first. For the next week, focus only on that particular emotion.

Most Diet Feelers report that when they really start to pay attention to a behavior they are trying to change, they recognize that the behavior seems to happen automatically, at a sub-conscious level. This means that, when they were able to stop or divert the behavior in the past, that they *really* had to give an all out conscious effort to beat their trigger. But because life can be hectic, they were eventually caught "off guard," and, before they realized it, they had responded to an emotion with an old, bad habit again. This

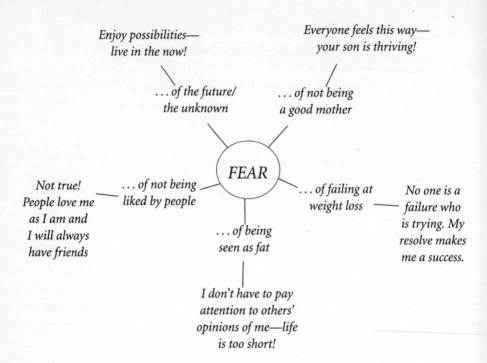

means that, in order to make a lasting change, an alternate, healthy behavior needs to take the place of the trigger behavior on an *unconscious* level. In other words, *you need to pioneer a new path...*

This means rerouting the connection from your emotions to your behavior so that, instead of your feelings leading you to an unhealthy place, that they lead you to a good habit instead. Brainstorm a list of things you could do instead of eating (meditate, read a book, exercise, talk to a friend, etc.) during those emotional moments and test them out until you find several substitutes you can incorporate into your everyday life. The idea is to find more satisfying alternatives to eating to help you deal with your feelings.

Once you feel you have a viable alternative to eating when your trigger emotion hits, use your imagination to integrate your new response at a sub-conscious level. To do this, start by imagining the circumstances when you might encounter a trigger; then, visualize yourself responding *not* by eating, but by engaging in your alternate, healthy activity instead. Imagine the new thoughts, feelings and self-talk that you experience as you participate in this activity. Vividly imagine as many details as possible about how you would act. Breathe the way you would breathe while engaging in this activity; hold your body in the correct posture. This mental rehearsal trains your brain to *automatically* act out the new behavior instead of the old one when you are faced with your trigger emotion.

You'll find that when you feed your true desires, nourish your soul, and fortify your sense of well-being, that your habit of reaching for food at certain times diminishes (right along with some excess pounds!).

However, remember that this process takes time; you cannot un-do firmly rooted habits overnight. Slip-ups are an inevitable part of the learning curve. Be sure to view any mistakes as opportunities for growth and understanding, rather than personal failures.

Focus on a new emotional trigger each week (or as long as you need) until you work your way through your list.

For extra help while you break your emotional eating patterns also be sure to...

Clear your environment of tempting food:
To give yourself an extra nudge in the right direction, clear your house, car, office, etc. of all the tempting foods you tend to gravitate toward during an emotional emergency. But don't panic; you don't have to ban those foods forever! Actually, the most effective way to change a food habit is to go about doing it in a way that does not make you feel deprived. That means occasionally, reasonably indulging in the foods you crave (especially the good-for-you foods). Just be extra careful that you don't indulge in response to emotions. And always, always, always keep portion control, moderation, and balance in mind (see page 218).

Stay present when you eat:
Much more than any other Diet Type, Diet Feelers have tendency to zone out and lose track of their food intake. They can eat half a pizza, and then feel the need to eat more simply because the food never registers with their senses. This not only decreases overall food satisfaction, but also plants the seeds for emotional eating by making "eating-without-thinking" a habit for you. Once you stop this behavior and learn to eat only when you are in fact hungry, you'll find that meals are a lot more gratifying.

Here's how to help yourself be mindful when you eat: the next time your body tells you it's time to eat (again, use the Hunger Scale for help), create or choose a soothing, non-stimulating setting to eat in. Take note: the less distractions, the better! Turn off the TV, put down your book or newspaper, shut off your computer, and *just eat*. Take the time to truly enjoy the experience! Focus on the food's texture and flavor and stop eating when you feel satisfied—don't wait until you feel stuffed. Eat this way as often as possible. Soon, you will be able to try eating with distractions; when you feel ready, test your new skill in a restaurant. When you eat out, it's often so easy to get swept away in a conversation or the bustling atmosphere that you can clean your plate without even noticing. Again, mastering this skill will take time, but with practice and patience (your Diet Type has tons of that!), things will eventually click into place, much like riding a bike or driving a car, and you will be able to eat consciously and carefully, no matter what distractions surround you.

How does a Diet Feeler pay attention to her health issues?

Don't wait until tragedy strikes to acknowledge your health issues. If you do, you'll not only lose years from your life, but you will also miss a golden opportunity for growth, self discovery and a life free from your food demons. Recognize that denial is a part of human nature and a very normal tactic that everyone (yes, *everyone*) uses at one time or another to deal with uncomfortable situations. Also recognize that dealing with your weight challenges will lead you through a mind-opening constructive experience.

~ GET IN TOUCH

- Get a realistic picture of your current health status and consider how your physical shape will affect your life, and the lives of your loved ones, in the future.
- Throw out the excuses and move from a stagnant state of denial and fear to a fulfilling path of self discovery.
- Optional additional reading: *Chicken Soup for the Dieter's Soul* by Jack Canfield.

Come into Focus

Begin by using all of your senses to really listen to your body and help you assess your current weight challenges. Diet Feelers hardly ever see themselves in a realistic light; that is, they rarely look as good or bad as they think they do. To get a more accurate view of your weight, take a picture of yourself, try on some old clothes, get on a scale, and consider how you feel when you walk up stairs or run vigorously. Also ask yourself this: can your present health status negatively affect your future? Be honest, and seriously consider how your current physical shape will impact your life (and the lives of those you love) in the upcoming years.

Next consider how your *improved* health would positively impact your future. Instead of concentrating on how your appearance could change, place the emphasis on your health and overall well-being. Reflect on how becoming the best possible YOU would benefit not only you, but the people in your life. For example, eating well and exercising could make you a better role model for your kids, provide inspiration to your friends, or encourage your spouse or co-workers to make a change. You'll also reduce your risk for chronic disease so you can be there for your loved ones in the long term. And you'll have more energy in the here and now to devote to the causes that are important to you.

After reviewing the powerful impact good health would have on your future, can you think of any good reason *not* to make a healthy change? Okay, if you actually were able to come up with an answer (or answers) to that question, it's time to. . .

Throw Out the Excuses

If you're thinking "I don't have the time" (*everyone* has the time; it's about choices); "I don't have the money" (exercise is free and fruits and veggies cost less than soda and junk food); "I'll start once I find a new job, boyfriend, apartment, etc." (you're waiting for a perfect time that may never come)—you're just making excuses. Your list could go on and on, but your "reasons" are just that—EXCUSES to justify your behavior.

So instead of making excuses, denying you're in denial, wallowing in guilt, or feeling sorry for yourself, try focusing on the future. Focus on a life full of possibilities and hope. That life is yours for living if you want it! Remember, you and you alone hold the power to make a healthy change.

If you feel overwhelmed and are unsure about where to start, don't worry, simply turn to your Diet Feeler Journey, page 134, where you will be encouraged to work through your weight loss obstacles at your own pace, so you can get the other side of denial and surmount excuses. . . and arrive at a happier and healthier, you.

How does a Diet Feeler win at social food struggles?

Since food is an integral part of socializing, your Diet Type needs to be prepared when you encounter a sticky (or maybe even a sticky bun) situation. Here's how!

⌇ GET IN TOUCH

- Teach yourself how to make conscious food choices in social situations by considering the big picture of your life *before* you make a food selection.
- Visualize potential social food weak spots and plan your other meals in the day accordingly.
- Find ways to connect with people that do not involve food.
- Optional additional reading: *Mindless Eating* by Brian Wansink.

EXPLORE SOCIAL SOLUTIONS

Just as you must do with all food triggers, whenever you come across a social food trigger, you need to STOP and remind yourself of your health goals. Social food triggers are especially dangerous because they are so strong. It is very tempting to give in to everyone else and shove the reminder of "I need to pay attention to my health and weight" out of your consciousness. Instead, take just a few seconds before you place your order, to go the buffet line, reach for a dessert, or make a food choice, to remember what's really important to you, and think about the best choices for you at that moment in your life. Only *then* make your food choice.

This process is not something you will do for a few days or a few months. Rather, it becomes an on-going part of your identity and actions. Women who manage to lose weight and keep it off for good, and those who have never struggled with their weight, are very conscious of what they are (and are not) eating, and there's no reason you can't be, too. Note: this will take a little more time for the Diet Feeler extraverts (ENFJ or ENFP) who are naturally more attuned to the stimuli in their environment (including food) and who are often involved in lots of social events, but with time and patience, anyone (yes *anyone*) can learn how to make *conscious* food choices.

Another social food helper is to visualize potential social trouble spots before an event, and plan accordingly. If you are heading to birthday party, for example, and you know your friend is making her insanely delicious and decadent double chocolate mousse birthday cake (and you can predict that saying NO is probably not a feasible option), then you can use the strategies of light eating in advance and portion control to help you out. Plan to eat light the few days before or after the party and then, when you arrive at the event, instead of trying to avoid the cake, you can have a smallish piece and still share in the fun. Plus, you'll enjoy the cake a lot more without the guilt. Remember to be mindful and enjoy every bite to the fullest!

Also, never make the mistake of showing up hungry to an event. That's as dangerous as it gets for your waistline! Resisting temptations, being conscious of your choices, and watching portions is ten times (maybe even 100 times!) harder if your appetite is raging out of control. My trick is to always have a high-fiber snack before a party, dinner, or other function, so I won't obsess about the food and can have fun with the people instead. And don't forget about the drinks in social settings. Cocktails can be loaded with as many hidden calories as that slice of cake—so watch out! (see page 212 for more info on making wise drink choices).

Finally, if even your best laid social food plans go awry, you can still take action *after* an event. Work out and be extra careful with your food choices the next few days, and always use the experience to get in touch with what got you off track. Don't let a slip-up start a downward spiral. Instead, turn these rough times into a positive experience to learn and grow.

Shift Your Energy

Explore other new and interesting ways to connect with friends and family that don't revolve around food. The possibilities are endless! Try something physical like a bike ride, ice skating or hiking. Or maybe a cultural event, like the symphony, the theatre, or a poetry reading. Join or start a book club, a gardening club, or a movie club. If a friend is feeling down, bring them a motivational book instead of cookies. Turn time together with loved ones into opportunities for development. Ask for input and ideas from others. When I was growing up my Diet Feeler mother would designate one day a week as "family fun day" and my sisters and I would take turns choosing the activity for the day. Trips to the library, historic outings (I grew up in Washington, DC), and museum visits were some ways we would bond and connect. On those days, food was always secondary to the heartfelt time we spent together.

How does a Diet Feeler stay motivated?

Diet Feelers are usually not motivated to lose weight just for themselves. Rather, they need a greater cause or someone they love to provide the "push." This means that Diet Feelers will often have trouble with self motivation. You will have a much easier time on your health journey if you know who you are pleasing, and who will be praising you, when you succeed. Since you thrive on positive feedback and social support, a Weight loss support system will have a huge impact of on your success. And the support and motivation you can offer someone else will fuel you with even more inspiration and enthusiasm for yourself!

~ GET IN TOUCH:

- Find a support system to help you on your health journey. The more health "buddies" you have, the better.
- Avoid health professionals who focus on a critical approach since the negative energy will stifle your progress.

BUDDY UP

The buddy system is your one-way ticket to a leaner (but not meaner!) you. Ultimately, health buddies are people who share a common goal. This might be a co-worker who goes to the gym with you at lunch, a friend you exchange healthy recipes with, a spouse you run with, or a neighbor who you take turns babysitting for so each of you can have time to work out. A health buddy could also be a personal trainer you work out with once a week, an inspirational mentor or role model who can guide you in the right direction, a registered dietitian you meet with once a month, or a weight loss pal you talk to online about how you feel. The more buddies you have, the stronger your support system will be because if one buddy is not available, you will have others you can turn to.

Your personal circle is a great place to start looking for health buddies. Let the people in your life know about your health plans and ask for their assistance. If they're not interested, no problem. Getting healthy doesn't mean you have to drop all your—let's just call them less motivated—friends, but it sure does offer a great opportunity to make some new, healthier ones! As a Diet Feeler, here a few things to keep in mind when selecting your much-needed support team.

- You're most likely to respond to a positive cheerleader type, rather than a bossy drill sergeant, *but* someone who doesn't ask anything of you and who tells you it's OK to eat an entire cake if you feel like it, is not going to do you much good.
- If you hire a professional like a certified personal trainer or a registered dietitian for support, find one who is interested in helping you as an individual and who will celebrate your successes. Avoid critical professionals since their negative energy will hinder, not help.
- If you join a gym, try one like Curves (www.curves.com). They focus on the woman behind the weight loss and offer a lot of support.
- Select people who stick to the basics of weight loss and healthy living; that is, eating right and exercising (see Chapter 7, page 223). Diet Feelers can be easily influenced by new "discoveries," magical cures, and products like herbs, vitamins, or pills that make weight loss promises. Be sure to stay away. These products are a lot of hype, but not a lot of help.

How does a Diet Feeler build self-esteem?

Self-esteem is your overall opinion of yourself. Women with healthy self-esteem feel good about who they are, and see themselves as valuable and capable. Women with low self-esteem, on the other hand, put little value on their opinions and ideas and constantly tell themselves they aren't "good enough." While it's normal for people to go through down times, sensitive and perceptive Diet Feelers are especially prone to focusing on their flaws and weaknesses and often engage in negative self talk—particularly when they are dissatisfied with their weight.

~ GET IN TOUCH

- Stop the negative self talk and build self-respect with positive affirmations (see Resourceful Self Talk activity, page 156.)
- Turn envy into motivation to make a change.
- Examine your personal relationships and identify and deal with saboteurs.
- Optional additional reading: *Your Body Believes Every Word You Say* by Barbara Hoberman Levine, *Emotional Blackmail* by Susan Forward, and *Pulling Your Own Strings* by Wayne W. Dyer.

TRANSFORM YOUR THOUGHTS

If you believe you are cursed and will always be overweight, or tell yourself you will always be heavy, then you will become your own worst enemy and your life will be a self-fulfilling prophecy. You need to recognize that the way you treat your body is your CHOICE, not your destiny. Instead of identifying yourself only through your weight *struggle*, choose to love yourself.

Begin by asking yourself how often you engage in abusive self talk like...

"I'm so fat no one will ever love me."

"I know I will always struggle with my weight."

"I should just give up, I'll never lose weight."

"I'm not coordinated enough to do this exercise."

"I always fail at this. Being fat must be in my genes."

Spend a few days consciously listening to your inner voice and keep a running tab of the negative messages you send to yourself. Note how many times in a day you put yourself down or tell yourself you're not "good enough." Next, review your list and ask yourself if you would say the same things to others. Would you criticize a friend, coworker or even a stranger the same way you do yourself? Would you judge someone else as harshly as you judge yourself? Would you discourage a friend or loved one from reaching their goals? No way! So why in the world are *you* being so cruel to *you*?

Realize that you shape your own reality by your internal self talk, and your critical, negative, and hurtful thoughts will drive your actions and set you up for weight loss failure. Low self-esteem not only weakens your self-confidence; it also destroys the self-motivation and encouragement you need for weight loss success. Good health is an achievement that is attained through one small victory at a time, and if you don't believe in yourself and cheer for yourself along the way, your path will be a hard one.

It's time to change your belief that "others are getting what you want" or that "you will always struggle with your weight" or that "you are special because you are surrounded by suffering and pain." YOU are special simply because you exist, and YOU alone hold the key to make a positive life-changing transformation. The next time you find yourself falling victim to destructive self talk, turn to page 156 and go through the Resourceful Self Talk activity. Use this affirmative internal communication to pull yourself into a positive frame of mind. Diet Feelers in particular have the keen ability of developing a positive mindset using this type of thinking technique. And remember, the more positive messages you send to yourself, the better!

Let Go of Envy

Low self-esteem can also lead to another diet downfall—ENVY. Have you ever seen someone at the gym or ran into a fit friend and thought "I hate how good she looks, I'll never look that." Those negative thoughts will also do nothing to help you on your personal health journey, and in fact will keep you from reaching your goals. How can you find yourself and your true path if you are constantly focusing on someone else? You can't, and you also can't "become" what it is you "hate" because your subconscious won't let you. Do yourself and womankind a favor and instead of competing with one another, use your Feeler strengths and turn envy into motivation. Embrace, support, and encourage one another, and instead of obsessing over what you don't have, work with what ya got and focus on developing yourself, your strengths and your health. Focus on being the best YOU, you can be. No one is as good at it as you are!

BEWARE OF SABOTEURS

Making a change in your life may evoke fear and jealousy in others who may subconsciously (or consciously) try to persuade and prevent you from following your new healthy path. You might have a friend who feels threatened by the strength and determination you possess. Or perhaps you have a family member or spouse who wants you to continue with them on a self-destructive path, rather than improve yourself, because they are fearful that the new slimmer, confident you will leave them in the dust. These situations are difficult for anyone who is trying to change their life for the better. But for a Diet Feeler, negative people can derail your self-esteem.

Honestly examine your relationships and try to identify the possible saboteurs in your own life. Do you feel nervous when trying to change your eating and exercising habits because you know that friends or family will make "funny" cracks and mean remarks about your new healthier behavior? Are people close to you "food pushers" who try to entice you to eat foods they know you are trying to avoid? Do they continually remind you of the times you have tried and failed in the past? Or do they get jealous or angry when you turn to your new, healthier friends for support and guidance?

As a Diet Feeler, I know your relationships are vitally important to you, but you have to look at them for what they are. If a family member, friend, co-worker, or whoever is not being supportive of your healthy changes, or even worse, are actually trying to damage and destroy your weight loss efforts, something needs to change. If you can get that person on board to support you, or even better, to join you on your healthy path (loan them this book if you have to!), good for you! Then you have transformed a saboteur into an ally. However, if your efforts to bring them around are ignored, or if you are continually met with hostility and anger, you may want to examine the relationship on a deeper level and determine why you are maintaining it.

Keep in mind that just like weight loss, improving self-esteem, disengaging in negative self talk, letting go of envy, and identifying and dealing with saboteurs takes time and commitment, but if you believe in yourself and in your power every step of the way, you *will* get there.

How does a Diet Feeler stop waiting for tomorrow?

For the Diet Feelers there is always the possibility of tomorrow… "I could start exercising next week, next month, next year…" But you could be reaping the rewards of improved self-esteem, more energy, and enhanced quality of life *right now*! So what are you waiting for?

~ GET IN TOUCH:

- It's your CHOICE. Don't wait for your life to change, take the initiative to change your life.
- Envision your healthy future and view setbacks as opportunities for personal growth.
- Optional additional audio: *The Secret of Creating Your Future* by Tad James.
- Optional additoinal reading: *The Secret* by Rhonda Byrne.

PREDICT YOUR HEALTHY FUTURE

Sitting around waiting for your life to change, for your passion to be ignited, for your soul-mate to be discovered, and for your weight to magically disappear, is just not going to make it happen. So instead of waiting for your life to change *you*, take the initiative and begin to change *your life*!

Visualize your healthy future and be realistic about what you want your future YOU to look like. In a world where model-perfect figures are paraded past us on TV, in the movies, and in magazines, it's particularly difficult not to let unrealistic ideals get the best of us, but setting unachievable goals will do you more harm than help. Choose a *realistic* inspirational image (perhaps a picture of you from a slimmer past, or an image of a *real* person from a magazine) and hang it on your fridge, post it in your journal, carry it in your purse, tape it your dashboard, your bathroom mirror, and your computer screen—wherever you are most likely to see it so it can act as powerful reminder of where you are heading. This image will provide you with motivation and encouragement.

TURN TOMORROW INTO TODAY

While envisioning your healthy future is a positive and impactful way to motivate you in the present, keep in mind that your vision can only become realized if you take some action each day. So start your Diet Feeler Journey and transform your awaiting tomorrow into today! Take your journey one day a time and remember when you get off track to take it in stride. Just because you ate a few too many Danish at work today, skipped exercising because it was raining outside, or pigged out at a party, that's not an excuse to wallow in guilt and wait until "tomorrow" to get back on track. Instead, revisit and reaffirm your goals and get right back on that healthy horse! Recognize that slip-ups are an inevitable part of the journey (and a normal part of life!) and rather than taking them as personal failures, realize they are opportunities for growth and understanding.

Part Two of Your Solution: The Diet Feeler Journey

Now that you've anticipated all the ways you might block yourself from success, nothing can hold you back! Let's develop your perfect weight loss Journey. The best way for your Diet Type to lose the weight and to keep it off, is by changing your habits, one introspective step at a time. This three phase plan will give you the time you need to **get in touch** with your personal roadblocks and motivators, allowing you to **discover** the insights and pathways you need to reach your goals and to **transform** the way you eat, drink and live so you can look and feel your best—all while **celebrating** your successes!

You and you alone hold the key to opening the door to a healthier you, so unlock that door and start walking! Take the path one step at a time and allow room for exploration and growth. If you take a few steps back from time to time, learn from them, and then start stepping forward again. Remember, this is not a diet you go "on" or "off" but rather an ongoing, improved way of eating, exercising, and living. It's time you realize your weight doesn't have to be a lifelong struggle. By using your strengths to build better habits that will last a lifetime, you will end the struggle, and start leading a healthier, happier life.

Overview
Phase One

Duration: At your own pace.

GET IN TOUCH: With what will motivate you to lose weight.

DISCOVER: The fundamentals of healthy eating and living.

TRANSFORM: Your diet—Think before you drink.

CELEBRATE: Your success!

Phase Two

Duration: At your own pace.

GET IN TOUCH: With why you struggle with your weight.

DISCOVER: The Joy of exercise.

TRANSFORM: Your diet—Empty calorie overhaul.

CELEBRATE: Your success!

Phase Three

Duration: Ongoing

GET IN TOUCH: With how to adjust your portions.

DISCOVER: The importance of goal setting.

TRANSFORM: Your life—Make healthy living last.

CELEBRATE: Your success!

Phase One
GET IN TOUCH: WITH WHAT WILL MOTIVATE YOU TO LOSE WEIGHT

During Phase One let's focus on what will drive you to make a healthy change. As a Diet Feeler you have an amazing capacity to dig deep and uncover your innermost feelings and you can use this ability to help you on your journey to better health. Keeping a journal is a fantastic way for your Diet Type to get in touch with struggles, find inspiration, express how you feel, and explore possibilities and solutions. During Phase One, take the time to create or find a journal that fits you. Whether it's a spiral notebook, a leather-bound book, a decorated binder, or a pad of recycled paper, use a journal that feels good in your hands and expresses your personality. Maybe your journal will include inspirational quotes or motivating weight loss stories clipped from magazines. Or you might include some of your favorite healthy recipes as well as pictures of friends and family.

Your journal will be as unique as you are and should include whatever will inspire and encourage you to continue down your healthy path.

Envision Your Destination
Once you have selected your journal it's time to dynamically consider your motivations for losing weight. Ask yourself this question, "What's your motive to be healthy?"

To begin (if you haven't already), set aside some quiet reflective time to think about the reasons you want to lose weight. Your first exploration assignment is to create a general statement of your weight loss goal in your journal. You may find this assignment effortless and say to yourself, "That's easy, I want to lose 30 pounds." However, when surveyed, many Diet Feelers had a different goal in mind than just dropping pounds—one that goes beyond the initial weight loss, to the desire underneath. Here are some examples:

"I want to…"

"Feel better emotionally and physically."

"Feel more energetic, attractive and healthy."

"Have more energy to play with my kids."

"Look in the mirror and feel good about myself and know I am the best I can be."

If you already have a firm grasp on your overall goal, go ahead and write it in your journal. Otherwise, take the time to brainstorm several ideas and select the one that best fits your aspiration. You can always adjust it later as you travel along.

After you have created a general statement of your goal, the next step is to clarify your motivations or purpose for achieving your desired goal. Clarifying your purpose provides the stimulation to keep you headed in the direction of your destination, especially on the occasions when you may get a bit sidetracked. Keeping your goal in mind, ask yourself the question, *"and what will that do?"*

For instance, if we stick with the first mentioned goal: Lose 30 pounds… and answer the question *"and what will that do?"* A typical response may be, "I'll feel better." Then ask again, *"and what will that do?"* One might say, "I'll have the energy to do the things I love."

Keep asking the question until you either run out of answers or fill the page with your responses. Whether you come up with 3 responses or 30, rest assured in the days and weeks to come you will spontaneously get the desire to add something else to the list. The idea may pop into your head in the middle of a work project, or occur to you upon waking in the morning. Whenever it may be, pay attention, and trust your intuition. The thought obviously means something or it wouldn't have come to your mind. Write it down, no matter how irrelevant it may seem at the time.

Take some time to review your answers and consider what they say about your life. Are your intimate relationships, professional pursuits, or friendships dragging you down or pushing you forward? Do you need to make a change in other parts or your life to help support your health and weight loss goals? Are your motives in line with what *you* want or with what others want you to be? Keep in mind that losing weight will not fix every problem in your life, guarantee a boyfriend or a better relationship, or bring ultimate happiness. Changing your life for the positive, however, *will* give you the vision and the clarity you need to reach your goals—especially your weight loss goals. More than any other Diet Type, as a Feeler it's important for you to look at the larger picture of your life as you start making daily diet and activity changes.

⁓ DESCRIBING THE _____ YOU!

Once you are clear on the reasons you want to lose weight, it is empowering to visualize the "new" you. Now to clarify, I just used the word "new" as a filler. In the following thought-provoking exercise you will be the one filling in the blank with a descriptor that is motivating to you. Let me explain. You will be describing the future "you" that will be uncovered when you peel away the pounds to reveal the "you" underneath. Will this be a "fit" you, a "healthy" you, an "empowered," or "vivacious" you? Find a word to fill in the blank. After you find a descriptor that feels right to you, answer the following questions with your future "you" in mind.

1. How does the _____ you look? Describe also the clothes you wear and how you carry yourself.

2. How does the _____ you feel about yourself and the way you look?

3. What are some adjectives that describe the _____ you?

4. What are some of the attributes that others use to describe the _____ you?

5. How does the _____ you feel about eating? While you are eating? After you have eaten?

6. Describe the energy level of the _____ you.

7. How often does the _____ you exercise? How do you feel about exercising?

8. How does the _____ you feel socially?

9. Describe any prevalent thoughts the _____ you has.

10. Record any additional thoughts you have about the _____ you.

Once you have finished this activity. Put the whole picture together and imagine the _____ you. Realize the ways you are already this person right now. Continue to focus on this picture of yourself in preparation of when you decide to reveal this part of you to the rest of the world!

DISCOVER: The fundamentals of healthy eating and living

Read Part One of the Basics in Chapter 7. During Phase One you will begin to educate yourself about the basics of nutrition and weight loss. This a crucial part of your journey considering the endless supply of contradictory diet and health books on the market today, as well as the influx of confusing nutrition advice, and the plethora of diet pills, patches, gimmicks that can make it nearly impossible for women to separate weight loss fact from fiction. Since your Diet Type can be easily swayed by new discoveries and is particularly prone to believing in miracle weight loss formulas, you'll want to take the time to remember that lifelong weight loss is not about going "on" or "off" a diet but rather about incorporating permanent healthy behaviors into your lifestyle.

The Basics in Part One are a trustworthy source of scientifically and nutritionally sound food facts presented in an easy-to-understand format. You'll learn the real basics about weight loss including the importance of portion control, balance, and the ins and outs of staying healthy and fit, *and* enjoying food. If you already have a solid nutrition knowledge base, use this information as a refresher.

During Phase One don't feel any pressure to drastically change your diet. Make whatever changes you feel comfortable with, and just focus your energy on transforming one aspect of your diet—what you drink.

TRANSFORM: YOUR DIET—THINK BEFORE YOU DRINK
Uncover hidden calories: Liquid calories are hiding in your coffee drinks, your cocktails, your sodas, your fruit smoothies, and even in your "hydrating" sports drinks. Instead of overhauling your diet in one fell swoop, your Diet Type has great success when making changes one aspect at a time—and changing what you drink is an easy way to positively impact your diet. Calorie-laden drinks may quench your thirst, but they won't fill you up and satisfy your hunger as well as the calories from solid foods. And the calories in drinks add up FAST. Take a look:

12 ounce glass of juice with breakfast: 170 calories

16 ounce café latte with whole milk for a snack: 260 calories

16 ounce sweetened iced tea with lunch: 120 calories

12 ounce fruit smoothie for afternoon snack: 300 calories

8 ounce glass of red wine with dinner: 170 calories

Total Hidden Calories: 1,200 calories

That's a *huge* dent in your daily calorie 1,600 weight loss quota. Identify and free yourself from the hidden liquid influences in your diet, and you'll drop pounds without even trying! In general, you should try to leave the calories to food, with the exception of nutrient-dense drinks like lowfat milk.

Even 100% juice isn't the best choice since eating the fruit itself is better because you get the fiber, too. Instead of drinking your calories try switching to sparkling water with lemon, lime, or even a piece of orange tossed in for flavor. Unsweetened seltzer water is a great, calorie-free option, as are low-cal drinks like Hint and Honest Tea. Coffee and any flavor of tea are free of calories too, just be careful of what you stir in—Splenda is an excellent calorie-free alternative to sugar, and fat free half and half makes your drinks creamy and dreamy instead of fatty and full of calories. And don't forget to drink lots of healthy refreshing water!

Since liquid calories are easy to overlook, it helps to track what you drink in your journal to find how many calories your beverages are actually adding to your own diet. Keep track of your drink calories for at least a week so you can get a clear picture of your drinking habits. Keep in mind that calories listed on product labels are expressed per serving size, and more often than not, beverages include 2 or even 3 servings. Take a look at the below list of possible hidden liquid calories, and at the chart on page 212 for help estimating drink calories without a label.

～ LIQUID CALORIE HIDING PLACES

Juice
Coffee drinks (including lattes, cappuccinos, and coffee with sugar, cream or milk)
Smoothies
Sports drinks
Alcoholic drinks
• Beer
• Wine
• Liquor
• Cocktails
Tea drinks (with sugar, cream or milk)
Soda
Milk and milk drinks
Lemonade drinks
Energy drinks

Once you uncover the liquid traps in your life, you can transform the drinks one at a time, one week at a time. For example, if you have a three-a-day 12-oz. soda habit (420 calories per day) experiment with other drinks that can take the place of the soda. Substitute this alternative for one of your sodas for the first few days, and swap out two of them for the next couple of days, and eventually convert most of your daily soda to your alternative (or water). (It's alright to have an occasional 8-oz. 100 calorie soda to tame a wild craving.) Use this same method with all the hidden calories in your diet until you are hidden-liquid-calorie-free!

CELEBRATE: Your success!
Starting a healthy journey is a major achievement and celebrating your successes along the way is a fantastic way to pat yourself on the back—you deserve it! A special non-food indulgence will not only help you stay motivated and focused, but also will raise your awareness of what you've accomplished. Start by giving yourself non-food treats for smaller successes (like a CD as a reward for starting your health journey, a manicure for reading Part One of The Basics, and a massage for cutting soda out of you diet), and save bigger rewards, such as a weekend vacation, for larger successes (like moving to Phase Two). The best reward is the one that will motivate you the most. Make a list of potential rewards in your journal, adding to it as you go along.

Focus on the positive, allow room for error and growth, and turn setbacks into opportunities to learn.

Take as much time as you need during Phase One and whenever you feel ready (when you have found what will motivate you on your health journey, examined the larger picture of your life, and transformed most of your unnecessary drink calories) move to Phase Two.

Phase Two
GET IN TOUCH: With why you struggle with your weight
During Phase Two, let's focus on why you are overweight or unhealthy. It's time to answer the hard questions. Are you an emotional eater going through a particularly bad time? Are you scared to lose weight because you

fear the unwanted attention you will receive if you succeed? Do you not take enough time to focus on yourself to reach your health goals? Are you afraid of losing the comfort you find in food? Are you unconscious of your food and drink choices and your daily intake? Are you in denial about your real size? Are you putting off starting a healthier path today, because there will always be "tomorrow"?

Use your journal to help you get in touch with your struggles and begin exploring solutions. Take a look at the below list of Diet Feeler weight loss trouble spots and consider how some (or all) of these things affect your own life. Review the issues and then rank them (in your journal) according to their importance and influence in your life.

Identify Your Trouble Spots:
____**Ignoring Your Own Needs** (page 109)
Are you are pushing aside your own health needs to attend to the needs of others? Do you ignore your own health goals to focus on "bigger" causes?

____**Emotional Eating** (page 110)
Do emotions trigger your eating more than the actual physical sensation of hunger? Are you using to food to help you deal with how you feel?

____**Denial of Your Health Issues** (page 111)
Are you in denial about your weight or health issues? Is your poor health impeding your ability to be YOU?

____**Social Food Struggles** (page 111)
Do you use food to connect and bond with others? Do social events wreak havoc on your health goals?

____**Trouble Staying Self-Motivated** (page 112)
Do you have trouble sticking with your exercise and diet changes?

____**Low Self-Esteem** (page 113)
Is your weight struggle a part of your identity? Does your negative self image impair you from reaching your goals?

____**Waiting for "Tomorrow"** (page 113)
Do you put off making healthy choices today because you figure there is always tomorrow?

Start with the one you rank as the most important, and then work through the advice, one at a time, gradually gaining the insight, understanding, and tools you need for success. Discovering and admitting to yourself what is really at the root of your struggles—and realizing that you do in fact have the power to make a change—might seem frightening at first, but you will soon find this process enlightening and freeing. Call on your inner strength, and recognize that with time, patience, and honesty, you'll find a new "you" emerging as you make peace with yourself and your health desires, needs and strategies. As a Diet Feeler this is a crucial part of your journey and it will lay the foundation for your healthy future.

DISCOVER: The joy of exercise

Read Part Two of the Basics in Chapter 7. If there were a magic elixir you could drink on a daily basis that would provide flowing energy and vitality, strength, stamina, sensuality, weight control, stress relief, muscle flexibility, clarity of thought, centeredness, and peace of mind—would you drink it? I imagine your answer is a resounding YES!

That magical elixir is exercise. (If you get a gut wrenching response to even hearing the word "exercise", definitely read on). Those that have discovered its miraculous effects consume it eagerly day after day. They don't need to force themselves, convince themselves, nor begrudge the time spent. In fact, they cherish and look forward to being able to rejuvenate their energy and renew their well-being. You may ask, "Who are these women?" These are the women that have found movement activities they truly enjoy. Activities that express a part of them. Activities that bring intrinsic fulfillment and physical pleasure to their lives. And that could be you!

Your Diet Type enjoys not only engaging the body, but also the mind and soul. Many Diet Feelers find yoga provides a spiritual experience, as well as enhancing strength and flexibility, like no other form of exercise. If you want to start in the privacy of your own home before exploring yoga studios, there are videos and DVDs that provide instruction. This way, you can try each pose at your own pace. One of my favorites is *Sarah Ivanhoe's Fat Burning Yoga.*

What about dance? There are an abundance of classes from dance aerobics to free-form funk. One form of dance that many Diet Feelers are drawn to (including my co-author Mary Miscisin) is called the 5 Rhythms or a Moving Meditation created by Gabriel Roth (www.gabrielleroth.com). More drawn to fitness centers or health clubs? *Curves* is an all-women center where you can exercise and chat with others along the way. It is a friendly, female atmosphere that encourages socialization during work outs. When it comes to lifting weights, a personal trainer is always a plus. They provide one-on-one guidance and usually some terrific motivational coaching as well. (See page 226 in Chapter 7 for a guide on picking a personal trainer for your Diet Type.)

The best way to find the activity, class or exercise program that is right for you, is to start exploring. Maybe you're more drawn to swimming, water aerobics or Tai Chi. How about nature hikes, bike riding with a friend, or team sports? Try an activity on for size, and if it doesn't feel right at the moment, you may choose to continue until you have established a comfort level with it, or put it aside and try another option. You may find yourself being mysteriously pulled back to that activity later (or not). Remember that exploring who you are and what fits you—the authentic you—is part of your personality. If an activity does not feel right to you, you haven't failed, you've discovered more about yourself and your personal preferences. Keep a list of possible activities in your journal, adding to it as you go. This exploration is as important as refining your eating habits—they go hand in hand. You'll find that the more you enjoy movement activities, the more you are motivated to eat healthfully to maintain your stamina and feel the joy of vitality of a body that moves!

TRANSFORM: YOUR DIET—EMPTY CALORIE OVERHAUL
Aim for abundance...
During Phase One you concentrated on converting and changing your drinking habits. How well did you do with this? If you drink plenty of water and eat your foods instead of drinking them, you have a great start at making sure the beverages you consume are not adding to your waistline. But now it's time to concentrate on what you eat. This may be where many women begin to fear deprivation and restriction. "Oh, no!" you may think, "Now's the time when I have to cut out all the foods I love!" Right? *Wrong*! Think "abundance" instead of "restriction." Abundance of nutrient-rich foods that is... and moderation, not all-out elimination, of the stuff you love.

One of the best ways to improve your health (and drop pounds!) is to concentrate on filling your diet with nutrient-rich foods—foods that are high in vitamins, minerals and fiber. The way to do this is to swap out the foods that are high in calories, but low in nutritional value, for nutrient-rich ones instead. As you learned in Part One of the Basics, nutrient-poor foods are generally high in calories, sugar and/or fat, but low in nutrients. They're often referred to as "empty-calorie foods," which can be a bit misleading; it's not that nutrient-poor foods are devoid of calories, but rather that they're devoid of nutrition. They dramatically increase the number of calories you take in, but neglect to fill you up with healthy nutrients—meaning that they do nothing to make you feel satisfied, improve your health, or decrease your weight.

Think about what you eat, and ask yourself: is my diet nutrient-rich? Is it full of abundance and nutrition? Will it make me feel better and put me closer to my weight loss and health goals? If not, how can I make improvements? Be honest with yourself. Potato chips (because they are fried) don't fall into the vegetable category—they're just empty calories. Even breads can be tricky: what does your sandwich bread offer you besides calories? If you're eating white-bread sandwiches, you're just getting more of those useless calories. However, if you switch to whole grain bread, you'll still be consuming calories, but you'll also be getting a healthy dose of fiber and nutrients, too.

Concentrate on eating real foods. This means that when you have to make a choice, think natural—think whole. Look at the food in question and ask yourself, Does this look like something that was gathered from the ground, picked from a bush, tree or plant? Perhaps hunted or caught? What has been "done" to it? That is, has it been sweetened, fried, breaded, or refined?

Using your journal, pay close attention to the empty-calorie foods in your life and how often you consume them. Are you snacking on vending machine cookies in the afternoon, but coming up short on fruit and dairy? Try swapping the cookies for a banana with some yogurt—the banana and yogurt are nutrient-dense choices that will fill your stomach longer than the cookies. Remind yourself: all you get from the cookie snack is calories, and no vitamins or valuable nutrients.

But, again, don't worry; you don't have to *completely* cut out all your favorite not-so-healthy foods (see All Foods Fit, page 218, and Craving

Tamers, page 262), but making nutrient-dense choices over empty calorie ones, more often than not, will help you cut out unwanted extra calories, and drop unwanted extra pounds. Use the 3-week plan below to guide you along your path to abundance and riches. If you need to take 2 or 3 weeks, instead of 1, to phase out certain foods, that's fine too. The important thing is that you transform your diet from empty-calorie picks, to mostly nutrient-rich abundant choices.

Week One: Phase out "junky" high sugar and high fat foods and snacks and highly processed "fake" foods. Phase in fiber-rich, natural foods and snacks.

Phase Out:

Cookies
Candy
Cakes and Pies
Chips
Doughnuts
Pastries
Brownies
Cheesy and Creamy Dips and Spreads

Phase In:

Berries and Dried Fruit
Fresh (or Frozen) Fruit
Fresh (or Frozen) Veggies
Popcorn
Nuts and Seeds
Salads and Greens
Low Fat Granola
Low Fat/No Fat Pudding
Low Fat/No Fat Yogurt
Frozen Fruit Bars
Hummus and Salsa

Week Two: Phase out refined-grain products and sugar-sweetened cereals. Phase in high-fiber whole grain foods.

Phase Out:
White Bread
Refined Bread Products
White Rice
White Pasta
White Flour
Sugary Cereal
Muffins
Croissants

Phase In:
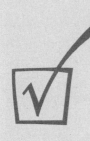

100% Whole Grain Bread
100% Whole Grain English Muffins, Pitas and Tortillas
Brown Rice, Bulgur, Quinoa and Other Whole Grains
Whole Wheat or Whole Grain Pasta
Whole Wheat Flour
Whole Grain High-Fiber Cereals
Whole Grain Crackers
Oatmeal

(Note: also see "How can you find the REAL whole grains hiding in your store?" page 208.)

Week Three: Phase out fried foods and unhealthy fats and large servings of full-fat dairy (a cup of cream, whole milk lattes or creamy salad dressings). Phase in lean protein choices, healthy fats, and smaller servings of full-fat dairy (an ounce of cheese, a tablespoon of sour cream, or a pat of butter).

Phase Out:

Fried Chicken
Hot Dogs
Pork Sausage
Whole Milk

Regular Mayonnaise
Fried Fish
Ground Beef
Hamburgers
Rib Eye, T-Bones, and Porterhouse Steaks
Pork Chops, Ground Pork and Pork Ribs
Large Portions of Full Fat Cheese
Partially Hydrogenated Oils
Fried French Fries and Onion Rings

Phase In:

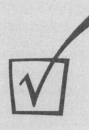

Grilled or Broiled Skinless Chicken Breast
Beans and Legumes
Turkey and Vegetarian Dogs
Turkey and Vegetarian Sausage
1% Fat or Skim Milk
Light or Fat Free Mayonnaise and Mustard
Grilled or Broiled Fish and Shellfish
Ground Turkey Breast and 90% Lean or Higher
    Ground Beef
Turkey or Veggie Burgers
Loin (like Tenderloin or Sirloin) or Round (like Top
    Round) Cuts of Beef, or Flank Steak
Pork Tenderloin or Pork Cutlets
Tofu
Reduced Fat Cheese
Small Portions (1 ounce) of Full Fat Cheese
Olive, Canola or Peanut Oil
Nut Butters
Olives
Avocado

(Note: also see "Plenty of Powerful Protein," page 209, and "Fill up with the Right Fats," page 210.)

CELEBRATE: YOUR SUCCESS!

Continuing to celebrate your successes along the way is an important part of your journey. A special non-food related reward will not only help you stay motivated and focused, but also raise your awareness of what you've accomplished. Continue to give yourself non-food treats for smaller successes (like a night at the movies for practicing saying no or a new outfit for transforming your daily doughnut habit), and save bigger rewards, such as a day at the spa, for larger successes (like moving to Phase Three). Remember, the best reward is the one that will motivate YOU.

Focus on the positive, allow room for times you may stray from your path, and turn setbacks into opportunities to learn and grow.

> Take as much time as you need during Phase Two and whenever you feel ready (when you have addressed your weight loss trouble spots, increased your activity, phased out most of your empty food calories and phased in nutrient-rich choices) move to Phase Three.

Phase Three

GET IN TOUCH: WITH HOW TO ADJUST YOUR PORTIONS

By the time you get to Phase Three you are well on your way to a healthier you! You know the fundamentals of good nutrition and weight loss, you have spent some time finding your motivation and addressing your weight loss trouble spots, and you've also changed what you drink, renovated your empty calories, and increased your activity. Way to go! At this point your pants should be fitting a little looser and your energy level should be a lot higher, but if you're hoping to shake off even more pounds, you'll want to consider watching your portion sizes a little more carefully.

While eating nutrient-rich foods will certainly help you feel full and drop pounds, if you eat too many calories of *any* food, you're still going to find yourself struggling to keep the pounds at bay. It's difficult and tedious for your Diet Type to determine precisely how many calories you eat, or precisely how many calories you burn, so instead let's concentrate on decreasing your portions and building healthy plates.

Plate Building 101

An easy way to adjust portions is to focus on what you put on your plate. Every time you make a meal, picture what your ideal plate would look like, and then build your plate from that image. Envision half of your plate filled with vegetables and fruit. By loading up on low-calorie and fiber-rich and filling produce, you leave less room on your plate for other calorie dense picks, and you increase your intake of good-for-you nutrients.

Next envision the other half of your plate and picture a mix of lean protein and whole grains.

If you are carb-sensitive, a protein lover, or just find it easier to lose weight eating less carbs (see page 207), fill the other half of your plate with ⅔ of lean protein and ⅓ of whole grains (see page 151).

If you are a carb lover, or just find it easier to lose weight eating more carbs, fill the other half of your plate with ⅔ whole grains and ⅓ lean protein (see page 151).

Finally, even though your plate is now full, imagine adding some fat to your plate. Because your plate is full there is only room for a little fat to fit, but it is very important that you do so. Fat not only adds flavor to your meal and helps you feel satisfied, it is also needed for many, many critical bodily functions. Throw some olive oil onto your salad, add a little butter on your veggies, top your potato with a tablespoon of sour cream, or toss a handful of nuts onto your cereal—you get the idea.

Keep in mind that while it's better to go hog wild with the half of your plate that is full of veggies and fruit, be sure to keep you lean protein and whole grain portions reasonable. Check out the Be Careful of Portion Distortion info on page 217 in Chapter 7 just to be sure your portions are appropriate for you, and not a 17 year old growing teenage boy! Also, in Chapter 8 you'll find a bunch of delicious and nutritious meals that have already been built for you (see page 239) as well as some ideas for snacks and Craving Tamers. For more help planning meals, see page 53, The Diet Planner Plan, for a structured approach, and see page 92, the Diet Player Strategy for an unstructured approach.

But first it's time to set some goals...

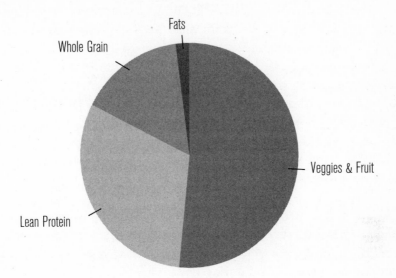

CARB-SENSITIVE/PROTEIN-LOVER

Fats
Whole Grain
Veggies & Fruit
Lean Protein

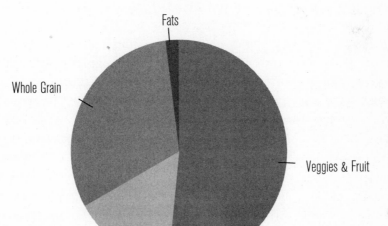

CARB-LOVER

Fats
Whole Grain
Veggies & Fruit
Lean Protein

DISCOVER: THE IMPORTANCE OF GOAL SETTING

Read Parts Three and Four of the Basics in Chapter 7. During Phase Three it's time to debunk some diet myths and set some realistic and attainable goals! In Part Three of the Basics you'll learn the enlightening truths to some of today's common Diet Myths and in Part Four you'll use a reliable means for figuring out a healthy weight for you. You'll learn the healthy and sustainable rate of weight loss, you'll learn the benefit of setting mini goals, and you'll learn how to turn your scale into your friend to help you achieve your goals and maintain your weight. Considering the number one reason women throw in the weight loss towel is because they get fed up when they don't lose the fat as fast as they thought they would, this is a very important part of your journey.

TRANSFORM: YOUR LIFE—MAKE HEALTHY LIVING LAST

Make a lifelong commitment: During Phase One you transformed the way you drink, during Phase Two you transformed your empty calories into nutrient-rich choices, and during Phase Three it's time to transform all you have learned into a lasting change. As you continue focusing on portion adjustment, building healthy meals, and dropping pounds, consider the big picture of your journey. Consider all you have learned about yourself, about nutrition, and about food, exercise, and making healthy choices. Consider what has worked for you, what has not, what you're still struggling to overcome, and what you can do to help yourself move forward and stay dedicated to your healthy lifestyle.

Keep in mind that, although this exploration is something you'll start in Phase Three, it certainly won't end there. Recognize that your life, as well as your weight loss stressors and solutions, will change and grow as you do, and this type of inner-reflection and resolution setting will change and grow too. The important thing is to consistently stay tuned into your inner voice, and to handle your health as you would a child you are raising. Your health needs just as much attention, guidance, understanding, and forgiveness, and you have to love yourself enough to stay on your healthy path—forever.

CELEBRATE: YOUR SUCCESS!

Continue to give yourself non-food treats for smaller successes (like a pedicure for accomplishing your first weight loss goal), and save bigger rewards for larger successes (like a cruise for getting to your ultimate weight loss goal!).

Focus on the positive, allow room for error and growth, and turn setbacks into opportunities to learn.

> Take as much time as you need during Phase Three to reach your weight loss goals. Once you have arrived at your weight loss destination, continue to use your knowledge and your skills to maintain your weight, eat a healthy diet, exercise, and live a happy, fulfilling life. This is not the end of your journey; it's the beginning of your healthy life!

ACTIVITY
Make Friends with "No"*

If I asked the following questions, how would you answer?

- Are your eyes green?
- Do you own a car?
- Do you have a cat?

All of these questions require a simple "Yes" or "No" answer, right? Now consider how you would answer the following questions:

- Mom would be so happy if you ate a piece of her pie. You want a piece, don't you?
- Everyone is going out after work. Can't you skip your exercise tonight?
- All the girls are coming over for a cookie exchange, do you want to come?

"No" is such a small word, just two letters... but sometimes saying "no" is so hard for Diet Feelers! Being of help to those you love and care about is the very essence of a Diet Feelers being. Though generosity is certainly healthy and rewarding, there is a big difference between caring and losing yourself in the wishes or demands of another person. When other people's priorities take on more significance than your own and you find yourself saying "yes" *when you really want to say* "no," you'll know that you have crossed the line from kindness to soul-sapping sacrifice.

So why can "no" be such a hard word to say or hear? The answer is fear—the fear of loss of love, the fear that someone won't like you, the fear that you will disappoint, the fear that someone will get angry. Understand that saying "yes" out of a feeling of fear, obligation, or guilt is a rejection of your true wishes and desires. And, if done repeatedly, "yes syndrome" can lead a Diet Feeler to constantly and unwaveringly consider other peoples' feeling *before* she considers her own.

So how does one start this process of making "no" your buddy? You'll first need to hear it and say it until you realize that "no" is not a big scary monster that is going to make other people hate you; in fact, the act of saying "no" is more like a little dust bunny! Furthermore, "no" can be your friend. So let's get to know this thing called "no."

Hearing "No"

When another person tells us "no," it is often simply because he or she is setting a limit, stating a preference, or giving an opinion. However, for many Diet Feelers it is the same as being told "You're a bad person, how dare you ask!" Help yourself understand that, overall, "no" is a simple *statement of fact* and has no judgment associated with it. (The only judgment that occurs is in your mind, and is based on assumptions about what the other person is thinking. "They must think I'm a jerk for asking. . .")

Asking for "No" Exercise   ·

Purposefully asking for a "no" response will help take the emotional charge off the word. In trainings, we had a great time with this exercise—it was hilarious to hear the creative ways people got another person to tell them "no." Your assignment is to get at least one "no" response to a request you have made on day one, two "no" responses on day two, all the way up to seven "no" responses on day seven. Have fun! Be creative! The only rule is that the other person cannot be told that you are doing it as an exercise. For example, you can't go up to your friend and say, "Hi Sally, I have to do this silly exercise to make you say no. Can I have $500?" Below are some examples to get you started:

- Ask a co-worker if they want to come into the office over the weekend.
- Ask your significant other or friend if they would like it if you shaved your head.

The more you hear it, the more "no" will land without the emotional impact, and many people have said this exercise even made "no" fun to hear. As you continue to do this, you will find your fears diminish and, with that, feel there is more "elbow room" in your life to act freely.

Saying "No"

As you learned in the above exercise, when people say "no" to a request, they are simply stating their boundaries—in other words, what they will or won't accept. Constantly saying "yes" to requests so that you won't disappoint others is at best emotionally dishonest and, at worst, wears away at your sense of what it is you really want, and compromises your ability to take your own preferences into account for even the slightest things. The only solution is to find your boundaries, and practice saying "no" when someone pushes up against them. Be prepared to hear how "mean you are" or how much you "don't care." It is a well-known fact that people resist change, and others in your life may react negatively when they hear you stating your preferences assertively. Keep in mind that you may not always know why you don't want to do something—that's okay. Often people do things they don't necessarily want to do, simply because it isn't worth the trouble to say "no." If you don't *really* want to go to a particular restaurant, see a movie, or stay up late—just say "no!" Any price you pay in emotional friction is well worth the return of your self-esteem. When a request is made of you and your gut, your head, your intuition, or any part of your being does not feel the request is in your best interest (for *whatever reason*)—tell the other person "No."

ACTIVITY
Resourceful Self Talk*

It's been said that "worry is a misuse of imagination." Our imagination and internal self talk have a powerful influence on our mood and what we may think, do, or say in any situation. These factors can make the difference between failure and success in reaching our weight loss goals. Simply put, when we repeat negative thoughts to ourselves and imagine they are true, we are programming our minds to *make* them true. If you think, say or believe, "I'm so fat, no one will ever love me" or "I know I will always struggle with my weight," you will unconsciously make these statements a reality. To attract something different, it is important to shift your internal conversations from what you don't want to what you *do* want. Use the following steps to transform failure, frustration and misery into success, satisfaction and joy... to create the reality you truly want.

Step 1. Notice your self talk: Write down any negative messages you have been thinking, such as:
"I know I will always struggle with my weight."
"I am addicted to sweets."
"I hate my fat thighs."
"I have a slow metabolism."

Step 2. Decide what you really want:
Do you want to lose a certain amount of weight? Is your goal to feel better? Look better? Are you simply tired of struggling with your weight and not fitting into your clothes?

Step 3. Use the P's of resourceful self-talk to make sure your affirmations are powerful and effective:

Positive: Make sure you create a statement in the positive tense. (Words such as *won't, don't, can't* are sure indicators that a statement is negative.) Instead of saying "I *don't want* to constantly struggle with my weight"

---

* copyright 2009 by Mary Miscisin, all rights reserved.

(which puts a picture in your mind of a constant weight loss struggle) make the statement positive, "I want to effortlessly maintain my ideal weight." That's okay if it seems too good to be true right now. Your brain will get used to the idea faster than you may think.

Personal: Although changing our own behaviors often has an effect on the actions of others, we must concentrate on ourselves. For example, instead of saying, "I wish other people wouldn't tempt me with sweets" (which is both stated in the negative tense AND focuses on the behavior of others), make the statement about you. "I" statements are terrific for this, such as, "I am in control of my choices."

Present Tense: If you state that you are *going to*, *will*, or *want to* do something, your brain will simply acknowledge the desire to do that something *someday*. Remember to think and act as if you already are, or have, what you want. Instead of saying, "I want to weigh 145 pounds" (which is stated positively and certainly states what you want) make it a current reality: "I weigh 145 pounds."

Particular: The more specific the aspects of success that you are able to imagine, the more powerful the ability of your mind to make it a reality will be. As you repeat your resourceful self-talk, involve as many of your senses as possible in the experience. For example, using the statement, "I weigh 145 pounds" you might:

- Visualize how fantastic you look in your skinny jeans.
- Hear the zipper glide as you zip them up smoothly.
- Feel the texture against your skin, imagine being able to breathe easily around the well-fitting waistline, bend easily, and pull them on and off effortlessly.
- Touch your flat tummy and smile at how wonderfully your jeans fit.
- Smell the hint of laundry detergent on your freshly washed jeans.
- Experience the confidence and satisfaction of feeling fantastic and beautiful.

Pressure-less: Relax. When it comes to positive self talk, the more stress and anxiety you put on yourself, the harder your subconscious brain will fight back. Think of holding a volleyball underwater. The second you let go and release the pressure, the ball comes shooting to the surface. If you try to submerge your negative self-talk by forcefully pushing it under with "positive" statements, you will experience a rebound when you stop piling on the pressure of positive thoughts. The key is to relax, believe, and be confident, and enjoy the process.

Practice: Keep your statements brief. Write them on index cards, type them, doodle them, sing them, or say them out loud. Use stickers, post-it notes or dots! Use them when you're exercising, driving or during moments like waiting in line. One Diet Feeler we interviewed bought a package of butterfly stickers. Her affirmation or resourceful self talk statement was "I weigh 145 pounds." She placed a butterfly sticker on the refrigerator door, her water bottle, her watchband, the rearview mirror of her car, the edge of her computer screen at work—anywhere where she knew she looked every day. Any time she caught a glimpse of a butterfly sticker, she would repeat her positive statement in her head, "I weigh 145 pounds." And she not only said the statement—she vividly imagined what it would be like to weigh 145 pounds, to feel it in the cells of her body and center of her soul. She felt a happiness and ease, knowing that she was metamorphosing (like a butterfly).

Soon, the butterflies "appeared" to help whenever she needed to make a decision. When she reached for a second helping at a buffet and, noticing the sticker on her watch, her positive self-talk kicked in and the associated feelings emerged in her body. She smiled and, instead of consuming a second helping, she felt suddenly, strangely satisfied with the first one. When she pulled into the parking lot at work, instead of looking for the closest space, the sticker in her rear view mirror triggered a thought to park farther away and walk a bit further. It wasn't long before she was carrying herself differently, making healthier eating choices and incorporating more exercise into her day. She practically bounced into work, feeling as light as a butterfly! Her clothes started fitting looser and eventually she reached her goal of 145 pounds. The best part was that she felt she didn't even have to work at it—instead, it seemed to come naturally, even playfully. What fun!

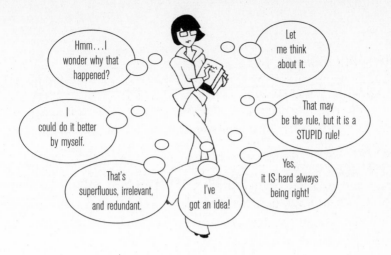

Inside a Diet Thinker's Head

CHAPTER 6

The Diet Thinkers
ENTJ, INTJ, ENTP, INTP

In This Chapter...

THE DIET THINKER PERSONALITY

- Seeks Knowledge and Understanding
- Objective
- Independent
- Witty
- Analytical
- Perfectionist
- Work is Play
- Problem Solver

THE DIET THINKER TROUBLE SPOTS

- Procrastinating
- Fear of Failure
- Rebelling Against Weight Loss
- Ignoring the Obvious
- Missing Other's Insights
- Trouble Staying the Course
- Using Logic to an Extreme

THE DIET THINKER SOLUTION

- How to Conquer Your Weak Spots
- The Diet Thinker Challenge

The Diet Thinker Personality

Diet Thinkers are typically analytical, conceptual and inventive in their quest for comprehension and understanding of the world around them. They live life by their own standards, and value intelligence, insight, and logic above all else. Diet Thinkers are constantly trying to figure out *how* things work and *why*. They are independent individuals who welcome challenges and are some of the world's greatest problem solvers. Determined, confident, and bold, the Diet Thinkers are epitomized in the characters Annie Sullivan in the Miracle Worker, Jo March in Little Women, and Hermione Granger in Harry Potter.

> **Diet Thinkers of Fame and Fortune:** Margaret Thatcher, Golda Meir, Marie Curie, Hillary Clinton, and Ayn Rand, all embody the characteristics of Diet Thinkers.

Because Diet Thinkers are so determined to analyze everything around them, they often find themselves getting lost in their own thoughts. Whether it's during her commute to work, while waiting at the doctor's office, or standing in line at the grocery store, the Diet Thinker is sure to use any spare moment as a chance for contemplation. Diet Thinkers are often drawn to the hypothetical and the abstract, and may postulate theories as to why something works—or why it doesn't. When sharing their views with others, they are accustomed to people responding with, "I've never thought of it that way." This is attributed to the Diet Thinker's knack for creative thinking.

When it comes to losing weight, Diet Thinkers will do what they do best, they'll think about it—*a lot*—sometimes for days, sometimes for weeks, sometimes for years. They are internally driven to understand the problem before taking action, but when they do take action they can be relentless in pursuit of the solution. Diet Thinkers may get irritated when an average "Jane" states she is perplexed with her weight challenges, for it is usually obvious to the Diet Thinker what systems were in place that led to Jane's problems.

Diet Thinkers in the Movies and on TV: Miranda from *Sex in the City,* Annie Sullivan in *Miracle Worker,* Ellie in *Contact,* and Jane in *Broadcast News.*

Diet Thinkers are extremely skeptical of simplistic, "dumbed down" formulas like: eat less, exercise more. They know that the relationship between food consumption and energy expenditure is much more intricate and complex than simple addition and subtraction. Since they are such big thinkers, they also see the larger scope of a problem—availability of healthy foods, mass production and promotion of junk foods, genetically modified food, food additives, misleading and inadequate labeling, food safety and global nutrition. Focusing on, and endlessly contemplating, the "bigger picture" gives a Diet Thinker ample opportunity to avoid confronting her own weight loss obstacles.

Research has shown that that an individual's personality has a profound influence on their lifestyle choices. Even more, these personality attributes are so automatic you may not realize their powerful affects—good and bad. To get at the root of your weight loss struggles, and discover the secret formula for weight loss success, you will need to take a long hard look at YOU. First, you'll find a summary of the Diet Thinkers personality's basic internal "instructions." Then, we'll take a look at what kind of unique mistakes this personality makes in the world of weight loss.

Read through the following attributes and "try each one on" for size and consider how they may fit your current way of life. Keep in mind that all Diet Thinkers are distinctive individuals, and we each have all four Diet Types within us to some degree, so all of the following traits may not apply. The most important thing to remember is that your goal is to explore and expose your personal weight loss barriers and drives, and to understand how to use your personality strengths for lasting healthy weight success.

DIET THINKERS AT A GLANCE

High achievers	Non-conformist
Knowledge	Wordsmiths
Objective perceptions	Principles
Independent	Enjoys complexity
Self-doubt	Authority independence
Intellectually curious	Architect of change
Conceptualizes	Systems designers
Competitive	Argumentative

Source: Otto Kroeger Associates www.typetalk.com

Seeks Knowledge and Understanding

❝ When it comes to eating healthy, do your research; buy the books, go to the internet and look for trusted sources of information.❞

—AMANDA, A DIET THINKER

Diet Thinkers have a voracious appetite for information and the ability to comprehend and use it. They recognize that the vastness and depth of what can be learned are endless, and it thrills (or overwhelms) them to know there will always be new information at their disposal. If they are interested in diet and nutrition, they will be relentless in their search for information—from books, to videos, to websites—a Diet Thinker can never have too many resources. They will explore everything from mainstream convention and research studies to alternative methods and the latest fads. Because they place a high value on intelligence, they want to know the information behind the information and love to draw conclusions, postulate solutions, and solve problems. Some Diet Thinkers learn by researching or observing rather than actually experiencing, while other Diet Thinkers experiment by testing their ideas on others. Although they definitely draw upon wisdom from the past, Diet Thinkers tend to focus on the future and on the potential of ideas.

When it comes to making a decision about their health, Diet Thinkers want to be well informed. They are reluctant to make a move unless they know it is a wise course of action that has been proven valid. This means they sometimes get caught in a cycle of never knowing enough, always discovering contradictory information, digging deeper for answers and clarity—and they can get stuck in an endless loop of analysis paralysis.

Objective

> 〔〔 I would like to control my blood pressure to be more in line with the American Heart Association guidelines and to reduce my BMI and cholesterol levels.〕〕
> —RACHAEL, A DIET THINKER

Diet Thinkers approach life and challenges rationally. They prefer to make decisions based on logic and information rather than hunches and emotions. Because Diet Thinkers are so "solution-oriented," and can effectively face challenges without becoming emotionally invested, their objective, stoic behavior can be misinterpreted by others as cold, calculating, or even uncaring. These ladies would not label themselves as "fat"—because "fat" is a *subjective* term. They are more likely to explain their current circumstance in *objective* terms by saying "I am 20 percent above my BMI." This objectivity leads them to view whatever is happening to their bodies as somehow *separate* from their daily reality, a problem to be solved... later. Furthermore, they may not feel an emotional attachment to their health or weight problem, which in turn may decrease their motivation to change.

Diet Thinkers rarely like to admit that they eat for emotional reasons beyond stress and boredom. They like to remain cool and level-headed and interacting with someone who is displaying intense emotions is stressful to a Thinker who is searching her databanks for a competent and logical way to respond to such illogical behavior.

They tend to rely most on reason, and logic, so when it comes to losing weight, they prefer to stick to a measurable goal, such as reducing their body fat percentage rather than a subjective goal such as "improve my self-esteem."

Independent

> ❝I don't like following diet plans. I just want to pick what I like from other plans, and do my own thing.❞
> —DONNA, A DIET THINKER

Of all the Diet Types, the Diet Thinker is the most self-governing (Diet Players come close). Skeptical of public opinion, they tend to ignore social conventions such as giving unquestioned respect to an authority figure. No matter how many titles one has or how highly they rank in status, Diet Thinkers still want others to prove their competence before they will value their opinion or position. As natural non-conformists, Diet Thinkers prefer to live by their own standards and they foster individualism and admire self sufficiency. So, when it comes to dieting, a Diet Thinker is likely to have her own unique definition of "healthy"—and their own idea of how to best achieve it. What may not appear to be a sound diet choice to others can be perfectly rationalized in the mind of a Diet Thinker because, after all, they are masters at viewing things from all angles.

Witty

> ❝I went on a diet—swore off drinking and heavy eating—and in 14 days I lost 2 weeks!❞
> —KATHERINE, A DIET THINKER

If you've ever been on the other end of a joke and wondered, "Was she serious or was she kidding?" it was most likely the sense of humor of a Diet Thinker. Diet Thinkers often have a dry, understated wit, enjoy irony and word puns, and they revel in their knack for sarcasm. In reading food labels, for example, with all the available nutrition information clearly listed, a Diet Thinker might say, "I miss deceptive labeling."

For the Thinker, humor is also used as a defense mechanism. They oftentimes use their sharp wit in order to "save face" and appear competent and in control. You can bet you are plucking a heart string when a Thinker rebounds with mockery or a witty comment. Let's say you mention to a Thinker that you noticed she's carrying around a few extra pounds. The sassy Thinker (who may feel embarrassed for not being in control of her weight) might rebound with "well, a few pounds is a lot better than the *few* brain cells you're carrying around."

Analytical

❝ The reason I would try any diet would be for health reasons and it would be based on medical evidence. ❞
—JULIA, A DIET THINKER

Diet Thinkers rarely take things at face value; instead, they like to examine the numerous aspects of a matter, debate many sides of an issue, critique any perceived shortcomings, and consider alternatives. One of their favorite questions to ask is "why?" They are hardly ever placated with the first response, wanting to delve deeper and explore further, forecasting trends and investigating additional complexities.

When it comes to weight loss, a Diet Thinker will likely start by analyzing the latest diet plans and fads. She'll pick them apart, finding every flaw and inconsistency before formulating her own ideas and theories. Then, she'll make charts of her progress and keep detailed diet logs and exercise records of her "diet experiment." This way, she has access to a constant flow of information, giving her fuel to do what she does best—think. The downside is, if her data doesn't support her hypothesis she'll likely just throw away the whole experiment.

Perfectionist

❝ If I cheated once on a diet, I was done. I want to do it perfectly, or not at all. ❞
—JULIA, A DIET THINKER

With a hunger for precision, Diet Thinkers strive to be the best and most competent in their areas of interest, with self mastery being one of their most compelling drives. Diet Thinkers set their own standards, and they have to meet them in order to feel successful. If they participate in something (including a weight loss program), they want to produce top quality results and don't like to make a move until they're sure they can deliver excellence. They pay careful attention to the accuracy of their words, the brilliance of their proposals, and the perfection of their actions. So when it comes time for a Diet Thinker to develop a weight loss plan, she wants to make "perfection" her goal—for better or for worse.

Work Is Play

> ❝ I don't enjoy preparing food that is messy to cook, serve or clean up because it unnecessarily wastes my time and energy.❞
> —KATHERINE, A DIET THINKER

Thinkers are thrilled when they can learn something new, solve an enigma or do something that "couldn't be done." They like to challenge themselves and their vocation often provides an avenue for this desire to be fulfilled. Working tirelessly with their attention focused like a laser at the problem at hand, often they "forget" that there is a world outside. Many will become so engaged in projects that they may miss normal body cues—like getting up to stretch, eating lunch, or even talking to co-workers. For a Thinker, this is pure bliss and their natural playground—overcoming a problem through the sheer force of their intellectual will and determination.

Problem Solver

> ❝ The weight management puzzle is simple, it takes 1- research, 2- implementation, 3- persistence, 4- fine-tuning, AND 5- follow through.❞
> —LEAH, A DIET THINKER

Tenacious and persevering, Diet Thinkers are intrigued and motivated by figuring out life's enigmas. It is irresistible for them to ignore something they feel is broken or needs improvement. They refuse to "make do" with inferior systems, products, and protocols when they know a better solution exists. While others may go along with the status quo and not question the order or value of things, a Thinker cannot help but formulate a superior strategy. For instance, in creating a weight loss program, a Diet Thinker may develop a system for charting the aisles in the grocery store so she can shop more efficiently, or she might design a lunch box with separate packets for each food group to ensure a balanced diet.

Their global approach may reach far beyond the immediate and obvious problem, as they recognize connections to the bigger picture or scheme of human destiny and universal progress. Ingenious and original, many Diet Thinkers are drawn to technology and the sciences. They enjoy hypothesizing about an idea, creating prototypes to test their premises, improving upon existing theories and devising strategies for implementation. One of the Diet Thinker's biggest frustrations is having a solution to a problem and having outside influences thwart its implementation.

WHAT WORKS FOR DIET THINKERS

Critical analysis
Devising their own best approach
Competition with self
Objective, long-range goals
Studying diet theories
Reviewing health and nutrition research

WHAT'S UP DOC?

Samantha's Story: A Diet Thinker

“ Studies that show there is a relation between weight and health are correlative, and as we all know, correlation does not equal causation. **”**

For some Diet Thinkers, discussing their weight is a battle of wits. It was definitely this way with Samantha. When the subject of her weight came up she rolled her eyes and let out a long sigh.

"You have to take this seriously," I urged.

She sat up straight, ready to take the offensive, "What makes you think I'm not taking this seriously? As I've already told you, there are no valid long-range studies that show my weight will adversely affect my health. If you look closely, the studies that *have* shown that the relation between weight and health is correlative, and we all know that correlation does not equal causation."

She sat back in her chair with a satisfied look, as if she had just made a particularly bold move in our "debate." Her silence and stare indicated it was now my move.

"But Sam, even if the studies are only correlative, are you willing to take that risk?" I asked

"I already know that rigid, structured diets don't work well, at least not for me. Anyone can do them on a temporary basis, but they don't translate into lifelong changes because they aren't flexible enough to fit into real life. I don't want to obsess over calorie counting and eating food that doesn't taste good. It's a waste of my time searching for diet food substitutes. That junk isn't even food, it's chemicals! I want to enjoy *real* food."

"Samantha, all the points you've made are valid BUT we both know that you are avoiding the subject. Regardless of whether your weight is causing your health troubles, your weight is definitely *affecting* your health. You'll agree to that, right?"

Samantha leaned back to carefully to consider her response. "I think most of the problem is that we are surrounded by an abundance of food in our society. We have such unrivaled technological advances, no one has to actually work or labor anymore. This doesn't even touch the issues surrounding our federal agriculture and food production systems!"

This intellectual debate was getting us nowhere. It was time to try a different approach.

"Samantha," I said matter-of-factly, "you are absolutely right, and I am definitely wrong." She leaned back slightly, appearing confused that I would give up so easily. In a very sincere and congruent tone I added, "Your health has obviously fallen victim to a vast Governmental conspiracy over which you have no power. And if you don't want to fight back, I'll understand and won't judge you harshly…it would take a very strong person to understand all of this and still have the willpower, self control, and determination to rise above these obstacles."

Like many Diet Thinkers, Samantha had fallen into the trap of thinking and debating about dieting rather than doing something about it. With such an all-encompassing world view, Samantha didn't feel compelled to change, because she could transfer all responsibility for her situation onto society. This position may or may not be factually correct, but it does place the locus of control outside of the Diet Thinker. To achieve success, all Diet Types must feel they have the capability and resources within *themselves* to effectively make the change, otherwise they fall victims to the whims of outside influence—as was the case with Samantha. I knew I had to break her pattern.

Abruptly, I stood up to end the appointment. Stunned, Samantha rose to her feet as well. As I walked her to the door I added, "You have a powerful mind Samantha, and it has served you well in many areas. You also have an extremely wise unconscious mind that is outside of your awareness, and it is constantly offering new and unique solutions to the challenges you have been having. Let me suggest that between now and our next appointment that you give your unconscious mind the permission to provide you with some new insights or solutions, and to institute a new behavior or two. I'll see you next time Samantha." As my nurse escorted a somewhat bewildered Samantha into the waiting room, I wondered what was going to happen at our next appointment.

At our next meeting, it was apparent that Samantha had been thinking deeply about a lot of things. I barely had time to sit down before she blurted out, "After the last appointment I was really mad at you! How dare you talk to me that way!"

"I had trouble sleeping for about a week, with your words going around in my head," she continued. "You *agreed* with me! That just didn't make sense, why would I be upset that you agreed with me? Anyway, one day after work I came home, pulled out my old tennis shoes and went for a walk. I haven't done that in years! Something you said made a difference, but I just don't *what* it was!"

Samantha ultimately understood she had been using information as an excuse not to act, and once she made that realization, everything changed. Over the next few months, Samantha made ongoing changes to her diet and exercise routines. She also began noticing when her mind drifted to blaming outside factors and learned to redirect her attention to what she could do in that moment to make her life better. With these positive changes, she is more than half way toward reaching her weight goals.

—Dr. Redard

The Diet Thinker Trouble Spots

A Diet Thinker's core value or driving force is a combination of self-mastery and control. Before they make a decision or take action they seek knowledge and understanding, and they trust logic above all else. Once they set their mind to it, they can accomplish virtually *anything* (including weight loss).

But once they have conquered their problem (including weight loss) they may slide back to their old habits; after all, they know they have the power or formula to accomplish this goal if they want to, so the challenge doesn't seem quite so compelling anymore. Just intellectually knowing they can do it is often enough for a Diet Thinker, and doing it in reality can seem redundant. With this in mind, it is easy to see why this Diet Type can struggle with weight and health issues.

Let's examine some of the Diet Thinker "trouble spots." Just as you did in the previous section, think about how, and to what extent, each weakness may apply to you. Given that you are a distinctive Diet Thinker, not every description will apply to you.

Procrastinating

> ❝I question not only the weight loss research but also who funded the research, how the participants in the trials were selected, and how the data was analyzed.❞
> —PAIGE, A DIET THINKER

When it comes to weight loss, the Diet Thinkers ability to analyze, digest and comprehend complex information is a real bonus. Studying the role of nutrition in the promotion and maintenance of health, and in the prevention and treatment of disease, is a critical step toward achieving an ideal weight (see Gain Knowledge and Understanding page 190). But all of that valuable knowledge and understanding won't help a Diet Thinker lose any weight unless she puts the information to good use. She can "think" about weight loss as much as she wants, but if her thoughts don't turn into action, she's just. . . procrastinating.

While Diet Thinkers pride themselves on their quick wit and sarcastic humor, they may find themselves using humor to aid procrastination by deflecting the emotional impact of their weight challenges. That's because when they are stressed, irritated, or feeling attacked or inadequate, they often resort to sarcasm and cutting remarks to avoid the real issue. They can be reluctant to discuss their weight because they don't want to admit their weaknesses or flaws (after all, it is already obvious by the way their clothes are fitting that they are not in control of their health as competently as they could be) and they abhor redundancy and stupidity.

Fear of Failure

> Once I cheat on a diet, I quit the whole thing. I never seem
> to get back on. My motivation goes away, I don't lose any
> weight and I get frustrated.
> —EMMA, A DIET THINKER

Wanting to always appear competent and in control, the Diet Thinker may not even attempt trying to lose weight if they have any doubts about the success of their efforts. If they start a diet, for example, but find they can't maintain it "perfectly," they're likely to get frustrated with themselves give up altogether. So, rather than account for a few slip-ups in their weight loss program, a Diet Thinker will rationalize that *not* trying to lose weight is the safest way to avoid failure.

While Diet Thinkers like to live in the world of objectivity (believing and relating to those things that can be measured and quantified), many will move to the world of subjectivity (paying more attention to their feelings) if their personal competence is threatened. For example, if they try to lose weight and fail, they may take this experience and expand, distort and generalize it to mean that they themselves are a failure, and then will vow never to attempt reaching their weight loss goals again. That's because the Diet Thinkers don't like the idea that food (or anything else for that matter) is "controlling" them. They will often rationalize that weight control is "irrelevant."

Rebelling Against Weight Loss

❝ Inside me lives a skinny woman screaming to get out, but I
can usually shut her up with cookies.❞
—ERIN, A DIET THINKER

Losing weight effectively is a complex process physically, emotionally, and psychologically. It's more than just finding the right diet or exercise... it's about finding the right attitude. Individualistic Diet Thinkers who like to go against the grain might find themselves feeling torn between wanting to look and feel better, and wanting to rebel against the social constraint that thin is attractive. When facing her own weight loss challenges, a Diet Thinker may respond with, "Who cares if thin is in? I'll *eat* what I want, *weigh* what I want, and *think* what I want, thank you very much. Who cares what the masses want?" Because Diet Thinkers are weary of conforming to social standards, they sometimes use this as a reason not to stick with a weight loss program.

Ignoring the Obvious

❝ It seems like dieting either consumes me where I think
about it constantly, or not at all. It would be nice to have a
balance and a happy medium.❞
—RACHAEL, A DIET THINKER

Although Diet Thinkers are typically quite reasonable, when it comes to their personal health, they may completely overlook how inactive they are, how much they eat and drink, how unhealthy their habits are, and what they really look like. Instead of using their typically rational way of thinking, a Diet Thinker may approach her weight loss challenges by employing softeners or subjective qualifiers to describe her current condition: "I'm a little overweight," "I'm just big boned," "My weight is fine"... come on, really? Of course, these softeners are a defense mechanism used to diminish the fact that they are not "perfect" in the area of weight management—which can be difficult for a perfectionist Diet Thinker to accept.

Because Diet Thinkers tend to search for a logical explanation for their weight challenges, they sometimes miss the obvious. Perhaps they have simply developed unhealthy patterns of eating and exercising or have a skewed perspective of "healthy." They're too busy looking for metabolic flaws, heredity predispositions, criminal chemicals in food, and conspiracy theories against the masses, to recognize how their *own behavior* is affecting their weight.

Missing Other's Insights

    ❝ I like to do my own scientific experimentation when it
      comes to cooking and eating healthy.❞
      —AMANDA, A DIET THINKER

It can be hard for others to point out a Diet Thinker's weight challenges because they're likely to take it as a hit to their competence. And because many of a Diet Thinker's defense mechanisms are manifested to create an illusion of competency, they end up hiding their poor eating from others—and even themselves. When it comes to taking advice from others, Diet Thinkers like to make sure it's coming from a competent, proven source. For instance, before a Diet Thinker will open her mind to the possibility of taking any weight loss recommendations from someone, she expects that person to live up to her own high standards. But since most people can't meet a Diet Thinker's high expectations, oftentimes she ends up rejecting advice and losing out on a different perspective.

Trouble Staying the Course

    ❝ I find eating health foods boring, unappetizing and
      cumbersome.❞
      —PAIGE, A DIET THINKER

Diet Thinkers have some serious advantages in the weight loss arena. The truth is, when a Diet Thinker decides to lose weight, and once she has the knowledge, tools, and mind-set necessary to lose weight, she will stop at nothing until she succeeds. The problem is, once a Diet Thinker KNOWS she can do something, there's no longer any need to prove it by actually *doing* it. At this stage of the game, the Diet Thinker's new, good habits often get derailed, leaving them susceptible to gaining back the weight they had lost.

Using Logic to an Extreme

" It is hard to find a logical, scientific diet that works fast."
—Rebecca, a Diet Thinker

Diet Thinkers, who value theories, ingenuity, and logic, are naturally drawn to the sciences. In fact, applying principles to facts to deduce objective conclusions and theories is what they do best. However, when it comes to their own health choices, this Diet Type will sometimes find themselves morphing science into science fiction. Diet Thinkers are extremely creative thinkers, so they can make a little information go a long way to support their not-so-healthy choices. For example, there have been several articles in the news that tout the "health benefits" of eating dark chocolate; a Diet Thinker may use this information to claim that if a little is good, then a lot is better. Using this extreme logic, they will justify eating three or four chocolate bars a day.

Diet Thinkers also don't want to waste their time or energy on things that are not important to them. For example, if a Diet Thinker is at a social event with people she doesn't care for or respect, she may avoid small talk by planting herself near the buffet. That way they can participate in a way that is independent from what they consider superfluous social interaction. Instead, they will make food the center of their attention.

WHAT DOESN'T WORK FOR DIET THINKERS

Weight loss groups, meetings or teamwork
Being told exactly what to do
Reporting to an authority figure
Discussing emotions
Following the pack
Focusing on just today

WHAT'S UP DOC?
Julia's Story: A Diet Thinker

❝ If I can't do it right, I don't want to do it at all!❞

When I first met Julia, she was 24 years old and moved with an air of purpose and determination. Extremely intelligent, she had just completed her PhD in engineering and had a high-ranking job in the Research and Development Division of a highly reputable electronics manufacturer. Although some might say she came off as arrogant, I found her confident attitude and tendency to question my medical diagnoses to be quite refreshing. With Julia, I always knew I would need to explain completely not only the condition she might have, but also the reasons why I choose one medication over another, the potential side effects, what we would do if the medication didn't work, and sometimes even the literature that supported my decisions. Frequently she would arrive with pages from the internet that described the condition she thought she had and, more often than not, she was right on the money.

Julia also had a wry sense of humor, and would often spring a word pun on me or share the absurdity in everyday situations with a good joke.

Not long after being promoted to the position of Manager over a division of engineers, Julia began to experience great stress. Handling administrative work and dealing with personnel issues instead of developing new technology left her feeling tired and drained; she did not like her new "people, people, people" job. Soon, her blood pressure began to rise and her weight steadily climbed. Her family became concerned and began to frequently offer her advice on how to remedy the situation. This only seemed to make the stress worse, for now she felt her home was becoming yet another place where she believed she had to live up to other people's expectations. "It would be a lot better if they just left me alone to figure this out myself," she said.

One day, when her weight had climbed to over 200 pounds, I reviewed Julia's medical record with her, taking the time to point out how, page after page and visit after visit, her weight had been steadily climbing.

I imagined that this factual information and irrefutable evidence of her weight gain would make a profound emotional impact. But when I asked if she thought about doing something regarding her weight, she only looked at me coolly and responded, "Yes."

I waited for what seemed like minutes for something more…but her silence made it clear that she had nothing more to add.

A former runner, Julia frequently complained that she simply "did not have time" to exercise, even though she knew it was important. She would resolve to exercise five times a week, but, after only making it a few times a week or missing a day, she would berate herself so severely for her slip-up that she would end up feeling even worse than if she had never gone at all. When I asked why she just didn't set a more realistic goal for herself of work outs three times a week, she responded right away.

"Because," she declared, "if I can't do it right, I don't want to do it at all!"

I asked, "Julia, do you have to do *everything* perfectly, or not at all?"

She looked me directly in the eye and said, "Yes."

It was apparent that Julia was approaching life as a Diet Thinker: one who has personal standards that are not only above *acceptable*, but also above *good*, above *great*—and even beyond *outstanding!* Her standard was to achieve "perfection."

I introduced Julia to the Diet Type theory, and the theory of temperaments outlined in the book *Showing Our True Colors,* and shared my list of favorite health and nutrition books with her. I offered that, far from being incompetent, Julia was actually a "perfect" Diet Thinker.

Julia was trying to do an A+ job at work, at home, with her family, and with her health. I offered an experiment: rather than getting an A+, she was to do a "perfect C+" job instead. If she found herself accidentally doing better than a C+, she was to readjust immediately and shoot for a C+. Julia reluctantly agreed to try it out.*

Julia returned in four weeks. She had lost three pounds! She had enjoyed the personality temperament research and eagerly analyzed various aspects of the health and nutrition information I had recommended. She related that, despite her best efforts at going for a C+, she was only able to achieve between an A- and B+ in all areas.

Through learning about her Diet Type and temperament, Julia became aware that her current position as Manager was not a fit for her personality type. After extensive deliberating, prolonged analysis, and carefully weighing the pros and cons, she transferred back to the Research and Development division she had been in previously. She said she experienced immediate relief at the move and felt like she was "home." Now that she was back in a job she loved that was more aligned with her innate preferences, her stress level plummeted, her weight continued to drop, and her blood pressure normalized.

At Julia's last visit she handed me a huge stack of papers.

"Hey Doc," she said, "Look at these obesity articles I found on the Internet..."

That's Julia.

*I credit Eve Delunas for this wonderful intervention—as described in "Survival Games Personalities Play" (Delunas, 1992)

—Dr. Redard

The Diet Thinker Solution

Part One of Your Solution:
How to Conquer Your Weak Spots

Here's how a Diet Thinker can "think outside the box" and beat those weak spots! Again, the matter at hand:

- Procrastinating
- Fear of Failure
- Rebelling Against Weight Loss
- Ignoring the Obvious
- Missing Other's Insights
- Trouble Staying the Course
- Using Logic to an Extreme

Read through the following Thinker-friendly solutions and decide if some (or all) of these things need to be addressed in your own life.

How does a Diet Thinker quit procrastinating?

Procrastination is knowing what you want to do, having the capacity and wish to do it, but still not doing it. Avoiding the very actions that will give you the results you want (in this case weight loss) defies logic, so you're probably wondering WHY in the wild world you do this. Here's the scoop (and no—it's not a double scoop of ice cream).

Our unconscious mind has the ability to delay or avoid doing the things we connect with fear. So more likely than not, you're fearful (gasp!) about making a healthy change. The thing is, we unconsciously train ourselves to unreasonably fear things simply by attaching pain to their meaning—and nothing has any meaning but the meaning YOU give it. So, in the words of FDR, "you have nothing to fear, but fear itself."

～ THINK IT THROUGH

- Analyze what you fear and push past procrastination.
- Turn your powerful knowledge into powerful weight loss results by taking action.
- If need be, take a break from work to strategize your health plan.

PUSH PAST PROCRASTINATION

Many people are fearful of making a healthy change simply because they assume they will have to completely overhaul every aspect of their lives. They think they'll have to give up all the foods they love (not true), train like an Olympic athlete (not true), and eat like a vegetarian (not true). Lifelong health and weight loss is not about going "on" or "off" restrictive diets, or making objectionable changes to your life, or subjecting yourself to eating foods that you detest. It's about incorporating healthy behaviors *comfortably* into your lifestyle. Behaviors that will improve, not diminish, the quality and longevity of your life.

Your challenge is to use procrastination as a catalyst to analyze why you associate fear with weight loss. Do you fear failure (see page 171), are you pushing against "thin" social constraints (see page 172), are you afraid it will take too much time and effort to get healthy, are you ashamed of your perceived inability to lose weight? Whatever your reasons, once you understand where your fear stems from you can *consciously* begin to unlearn this connection and start associating positive things to getting healthy as you experience success with your Diet Thinker Challenge (see page 190) and turn your thoughts and knowledge into action.

So instead of continually assessing how dietary components influence the health status in humans, incorporate a few more whole grains into your diet. Instead of reading yet another epidemiologic study about the positive health effects of phytochemical intakes, eat more fruits and veggies. And instead of endlessly debating the most effective type of exercise, the correct duration, the exact resistance and pace necessary, pick an activity and try it on for size and fit.

To start the positive ball rolling, instead of saying to yourself, "Tomorrow, I'll be good," tell yourself, "Tomorrow, I'll be bad." Diet Thinkers who do this report that they can be "good" for a day, knowing they can be "bad" tomorrow. What usually happens is they feel so triumphant and successful having made it through a good day, they do it again the next day, putting off being "bad" one day at a time.

Do the "Thomas Edison"

Any time Edison came up against a problem, he would take a nap...but take a nap in a very specific way. He would ask his unconscious (or collective unconscious) to come up with a solution while he slept. He then would free his mind and sleep deeply. More often than not when he awoke the answer would "pop" into his head.

A variation on this for weight loss is to put your problem on paper. Write out what your challenge is in detail (don't list solutions) and when the problem is ALL out, put down your pen and leave the paper in your favorite "thinking spot" (desk/office/etc.). Free your mind and instruct your unconscious to come up with a creative solution that it has not considered yet—that when implemented would be an easy and elegant way to overcome the challenge.

Excuse Yourself from Work

Many Diet Thinkers put an extraordinary amount of time and energy into their work, and have fun doing it. However, this concentrated focus on work not only makes it difficult to give adequate time and attention to other areas of your life (including your health), it also facilitates (yup, you got it) weight loss procrastination. It's time to excuse yourself from your usual responsibilities to concentrate on your weight loss strategy.

If you're a workaholic (you know who you are) take a complete break from your routine and take a few days off work (or at least a weekend) to concentrate fully on Part Three of your Diet Thinker Challenge (see page 190). Believe me, no matter how invaluable you feel you are, your job will survive a few days without you. Remember, your health, and ultimately your life, are at stake here. And how can you expect to work to your full potential if your health is down the tubes? If you don't have the vacation time available, see your Doctor and see if he or she will give you a few days medical leave. Dr. Redard frequently authorizes medical time off for these endeavors.

How does a Diet Thinker lose her fear of failure?

The bad news is there are no shortcuts, magical solutions, or "easy" ways to loss weight and get in shape. (Sorry, but someone has to say it.) The good news is, with the right information and mind-set you will lose weight—here's how.

~ THINK IT THROUGH

- Be objective about setbacks. Learn from your mistakes and get back on track.
- Listen to your wisdom and always make conscious health decisions.

Learn That Failure Can Equal Success

We all have had episodes where we did not completely achieve a goal we really wanted (like losing weight), and it is human nature to be disappointed that we may have fallen short. However, Diet Thinkers may take their less-than-successful weight loss experience and misinterpret it to mean that they are totally incompetent in this area, that even attempting to achieve the goal was stupid, and then vow to never attempt reaching the goal again. What happened here? This is a Diet Thinker being subjective (I'm a failure, that diet is stupid, I'll never get to the weight I want) instead of being in their usual state of objectivity (The scale shows I gained two pounds this week; that aroma of that pastry stimulated my appetite and my defenses lowered, I only exercised one time this week instead of my usual four times). Notice the difference in these two approaches?

How do you overcome this? BE OBJECTIVE about setbacks! Use your strengths! The road to achieving any goal is laden with challenges, road-blocks, pitfalls, obstacles, and detours, and the road to weight loss is no different. Meeting your weight loss challenges and learning from them is vital for your long-term success because these episodes offer valuable information on how to fine tune your approach. In fact, it may even be said that these mini "failures" are *imperative* to lifelong good health.

Taking each challenge, going through it, gathering and learning from the experience, and then applying the learning so you may avoid future challenges makes achieving your long-range health goals much, much more likely to happen. Diet Thinkers who lose weight and manage to keep it off don't beat themselves up and throw in the towel when they over-eat at a party, miss a work out, or have a bad "diet" day. They learn from their experience, let it go, and get back into a winning weight loss position. So whether this is your first try at weight loss or your fiftieth, when you happen to experience a "failure" know that you have been given an unprecedented opportunity to learn something new.

ACHIEVE EXCELLENCE

When setting goals, create different levels of achievement such as, Level 1: take stairs at work, Level 2: take 10 a minute walk, Level 3: do 20 minutes of exercise, Level 4: take an exercise class. Assign yourself a level to accomplish for that day, do an excellent job and reward yourself for your competence.

MAKE CONSCIOUS DECISIONS

Most importantly, always, always, always, pay attention to your wisdom. If you happen to stray off course simply yell "STOP!" in your head (or out loud if you are brave). Pause and analyze the circumstance, logic it through and conclude if the current course of action is congruent with your long-range goals. If you decide to indulge in a doughnut or skip a work out, you are not allowed to berate yourself, after all—you astutely made your decision, right?

How does a Diet Thinker stop rebelling?

If there's a part of you that wants to lose weight, but a part that doesn't want to, it's time to connect with the rebel within.

～ THINK IT THROUGH

- Make an attitude adjustment and get healthy because YOU want to.
- Examine what your emotions are telling you. For more information on how to make negative emotions work for you read chapter 11—The Ten Emotions of Power—in the book, *Awaken the Giant Within* by Anthony Robbins.

REACH THE REBEL WITHIN

I'm sure you have heard a person say, "Part of me wants this, but part of me wants that." We all have "parts" of ourselves that *appear* to want diametrically opposed goals. When both these parts are active, a person may appear to be in a push-pull mode with two captains running the ship. This is frequently the cause of *incongruence*—when you publically state that you want one thing but your actions demonstrate that you want something else. The way to remedy this is to get both "parts", or both captains, working together to meet the same goal—when you do this it leads to *congruence* in thought and action. To do this, pick an area that you have been incongruent—that is, an area or issue where one part of you wants one thing, but another part of you wants something else. Then directly address the "parts"...

Okay part ONE, what do you want? "I want to be thin because then I'll have more stamina and energy, I'll be able to think clearer, I will appear more competent and in control, I'll look better in my professional outfits, and people will take me more seriously."

Okay part TWO, what do you want? "I want to relax, not have to struggle or watch what I eat. I want to do what I want, I don't care about what others think about my body, they can go to hell, the brain is more important than the body anyway."

Then ask both parts *why* they want that, and *what* will that do for them. If you keep asking and asking, eventually you'll discover that both parts ultimately want the same thing... they just want you to be happy. With this realization what frequently happens is that both parts "shake hands" and begin working together to reach a common goal—a state of congruence.

If getting healthy and losing weight is going to make YOU happy, then you have nothing left to rebel against since YOU will be making the changes to please yourself! So tune out the social static (you're good at that!), create your strategy (see page 190), and get on with it. This internal struggle is causing you a lot more turmoil than need be.

REFLECT INSTEAD OF DEFLECT
The next time you make a clever crack about your weight or defend your "larger" size, instead of averting emotion, allow it entry and examine its purpose. What is the meaning in the message? Emotions erupt for a reason, they are messengers telling you to pay attention and take action. Your job is to interpret the signal, not block it. Ignoring the emotions will only impede logical reasoning (yikes!), weaken your confidence (gulp), and do nothing to help you solve the real issue—the fact that you are dissatisfied about your weight.

DO THE "EINSTEIN"
Einstein was famous for his "thought experiments"—also known as "what if" experiments. He would start out with a premise like "What if I could travel the speed of light" and then observe what would happen if that premise were true.... Relating to weight loss do a "thought experiment" such as "What if I achieved my ideal weight easily, comfortably, and permanently? How did that occur and what would be different?

How does a Diet Thinker stop ignoring the obvious?
Diet Thinkers, you can't attain "perfection" unless you are willing to be honest with yourself about your health and habits.

> ~ **THINK IT THROUGH**
>
> - Get a realistic/objective picture of your health and current physical shape.
> - Uncover your unhealthy blind spots by analyzing your habits.
> - Manage food triggers by resetting your desire dial.

TIME FOR A REALITY CHECK

If you want to "get in the weight loss game" you have to get your head in first, and getting a realistic/objective picture of where you are starting out is a really good idea. Step on a scale, take out the tape measure, get a body fat analysis, or go to your Doctor for an impartial objective opinion (see Know Your Numbers page 193). DO NOT ask your best friend or spouse "Do you think I am fat?"

UNCOVER YOUR BLIND SPOTS

Your unhealthy blind spots could be derailing your diet and your health a lot more than you realize. Are you skipping breakfast? Are you missing a multivitamin? Are you reaching for foods simply because they are there, and not because you are hungry? Are you snacking late at night? Are you eating loads of processed foods? Are you only eating once a day? Are you snacking between meals on junk? Are you eating a lot of fast food? Are you sitting in front of a computer 14 hours a day?

What separates the weight loss winners from the losers is that the winners have habits that are conducive towards success, while the losers have habits that facilitate failure. A habit is simply a pattern of behavior that is developed through constant repetition. If a new (healthier) behavior is repeated enough times, it eventually gets programmed into your subconscious and becomes a part of your routine. So what you need to do is analyze your life and identify your not-so-healthy habits, so you can replace those behaviors with helpful habits that will last a lifetime (see Analyze your Habits page 196).

MANAGE TRIGGERS

Many of us have urges and cravings for certain foods that seem to magically trigger us into stuffing our face before we are even aware of it. There is a simple way to break this trigger-eat response called "resetting the dial" (adapted from Anthony Robbins). While this exercise can be used by all Diet Types, it's particularly useful for the intuitive, problem-solving Diet Thinkers.

Do this for a moment—consider a food that you have had a craving for and would like to feel differently about. Consider that food, and on a scale of -10 to +10, how much do you desire it right now, this moment? For example, a +10 desire would be I HAVE TO HAVE CHOCOLATE NOW! A -10 desire would be YUCK, keep that away from me! A level 0 is considered neutral—you could take it or leave it. So what is your current level of desire?

Current Level of Desire _____

Now, let's say your current level of desire for chocolate is +5. Ask yourself, what would have to happen to make my desire a level +3? For some people it may be a brand of chocolate they didn't like, or having nuts in it, etc. Now ask yourself what would have to happen to make your desire for the chocolate a level -1 (slightly undesirable). Again, for some it could be that the chocolate is old, or partially melted. Now, ask yourself what would have to happen to make your desire a level -5. For some, it could be chocolate mixed in a food they don't like, for example okra stew. Now, go ahead and make your desire a -10 (go ahead, you can do it!) Imagine the chocolate crawling with maggots sitting on a pile of decaying garbage. Gross!

Ok, shake it off and come back to being here. Now, what did that exercise tell us? It tells us your desire for any food *in that moment* is how you view it in your mind's eye (this happens at the unconscious level for most people). If you want to break that craving, consciously go through the above process by ranking your current level of desire, and imagining what it would take to "turn down the dial"

How does a Diet Thinker pay attention to others' insights?

Thinking (what Diet Thinkers do best!) is often an internal process out of the awareness of those around you. While this is fine, natural, and appropriate at times, at other times it leads the Diet Thinker to miss out on valuable thoughts, insights, and contributions from others.

┌───┐
│ ～ THINK IT THROUGH   │
│   │
│   • Conduct a feedback experiment to reveal valuable health informa- │
│   tion from people you respect.   │
│   • Tap into the universal intellect with "perceptual positions." │
└───┘

Conduct a Feedback Experiment

For one day (and one day only) commit to ask at least five people you respect for feedback/advice about your weight problem. BUT, here are the rules. You must write out your problem/concern/question such that it has a specific answer (i.e.—it can't be an open ended question such as "what do you think I should do"—a closed ended question would be "What are three things I can do that would assist me in reaching my goal"... Open ended: "Should I lose weight" Close ended "How much weight specifically should I lose?" THEN predict what answers others will give you (this is your hypothesis). Now, go conduct the experiment. How did their answers line up against your hypothesis? The trend will usually be that they line up exactly—therefore you already know what you need to do— so go do it! Or, the answers will be completely something you haven't thought of—these are especially valuable for these answers have been outside of your awareness (by definition!). If the suggestions/answers are completely off base— then the source is completely off base, and that's OK. But frequently/often valuable new information will be revealed.

Try "Perceptual Positions"

Learn to tap into the universal intellect by doing what psychologists call assuming "perceptual positions" (Based on the work of Robert Dilts.) To do this, think back to a "limiting situation"—a situation where you wished you acted differently or made a different choice. (This could be when you "slipped" from your diet, failed to exercise when you wanted to, etc.) Got it? Now, do the following:

• Go back to your chosen experience in your mind's eye. Imagine that you are back at that moment seeing the experience through your own eyes, seeing what you saw, hearing what you heard, feeling what you felt, thinking what you thought—this is called the 1st position. Use 1st person language when describing what is going on—"I am seeing" "I am hearing" "I feel," etc.

- If there was another person present during this past experience, imagine now that you are "in the shoes" of that person looking out and seeing you. (If there wasn't another person present, you can imagine a coach or an infinitely wise mentor.) Associate into their body to view yourself from this new position—the 2nd position. Now that you are in the place of the observer and are able to see yourself, feel the things the observer felt, see the things the observer saw, think the things the observer thought. Describe the situation using 2nd person language—"You are" "You look" etc. Notice how this new point of view offers new insights.
- Now, view the past experience as though you were sitting in a theater and watching you and the other person up there on the screen in a movie. (This is the 3rd position.) From this separate, yet connected, position notice the two people interacting. Describe the situation with 3rd person language—"They are" "She is saying", etc.
- Now come back to the 1st position (Seeing the world through your eyes) while carrying all of you observations and learning's that come from experiencing other points of view. With this new information, think about what you can you do differently in the future to procure a more favorable (weight loss) outcome.

While this process is valuable for all Diet Types, it's immensely worthwhile to get a Diet Thinker (especially the introverted INTJs and INTPs) out of their head and experiencing the world through the point of views of others.

How does a Diet Thinker stay the course?

Just knowing you have the capability to lose weight is not enough to protect you from weight-related diseases, increase your energy, or make you feel good about your well-being. It is an undeniable, well-researched, no-doubt-about-it fact that a poor diet combined with physical inactivity causes obesity, heart disease, diabetes, and other diet-related diseases, and costs billions in health care and lost productivity. Instead of being part of this problem, challenge yourself to be part of the *permanent* solution. Ultimate success is not gained by getting healthy and reaching your target weight; it is reached by staying there.

‾‾

~ THINK IT THROUGH

- Recognize your goal is not to reach an ideal weight just to prove you can do it, but rather lifelong health.
- Develop new and interesting ways to continually challenge yourself to stay healthy.

_____

MAKE IT CHALLENGING

Challenge yourself to improve your personal best results. For example, if you run a few miles three times a week, challenge yourself to train for a half marathon, if you complete the half marathon, challenge yourself to run a full marathon, if you complete the full marathon, challenge yourself to beat your time. If you tire of your diet regime, re-analyze your life, and challenge yourself to invent a new, interesting method for success. If you get bored of doing the same exercise day in and day out, challenge yourself to change your activity routine—hike a couple of days, bike another, and play a game of tennis on the weekend. If you get fed up with the same old activities, seek out new activities and be willing to practice and challenge yourself to improve your skills—karate, ballroom dancing, yoga, Pilates, or whatever. As a problem solving Diet Thinker you should draw on your strengths to find inventive ways to stay in the weight loss game—for life.

MAKE IT INTERESTING

Employ new technology: Diet Thinkers are most likely to use the latest technological gadget to assist their weight loss and support long-lasting health. Pedometers, electronic scales, hand held body fat analyzers, heart rate monitors, 24 hour calorie expenditure monitors, computer exercise and calorie monitoring programs, hand-held calorie counters. The choices are endless.

Employ "old" technology: Don't discount old technology either. The old rubber band around the wrist (and snapping it if you're tempted) trick still works! If the display of pastries happens to be calling your name... snap that rubber band and walk away. One Diet Thinker I know carries a satchel of strong-smelling herbs that she pulls out and whiffs if her nose catches a scent of tempting foods. Use whatever "technology" works for YOU.

How does a Diet Thinker stop using logic to an extreme?

Do you justify eating large quantities of potato chips because you figured out the potassium content of the chips is higher than that of a banana? Are you excusing your daily indulgence of four chocolate bars because you read a study hyping the benefits of antioxidants found in dark chocolate? Do you avoid "fattening" carbohydrates, but regularly stuff yourself with a fatty steak or pork rinds?

～ THINK IT THROUGH

- Don't use science-fiction as an excuse to support your poor health choices.
- Seek knowledge from reputable sources and get the *real* facts before making health decisions.

LOOK AT THE BIG PICTURE

Get a grip. Step back and look at the bigger picture of your diet and habits. You may be getting potassium in those chips, but you're also getting a boatload of not-so-healthy junk including sodium and lots of nutrient-poor calories. And while *small* portions (about an ounce per day) of antioxidant-rich dark chocolate can be part of healthy diet, huge quantities (loaded with way too much fat, sugar and calories) will do you a lot more harm than help. And the truth is carbohydrates don't cause weight gain any more than fat or protein. If you eat too many calories—whether they come from carbs, protein, fat, or... hello!—pork rinds—you gain weight.

Instead of using logic to an extreme to excuse (ah-hem) your not-so-healthy indulgences, turn to your Diet Thinker Challenge and do what you do best. Seek knowledge and understanding from reliable sources and make decisions about your health based on fact, not fiction. When it comes to weight loss, science is on your side.

Part Two of Your Solution:
The Diet Thinker Challenge

Now that you've anticipated all the ways you might block yourself from success, nothing can hold you back! Let's develop your perfect weight loss plan. The most effective way for your Diet Type to take back control is to challenge yourself to be your own weight loss master—to inform yourself about what your body needs, analyze your current health and habits, and design and implement a weight loss system you deem workable. Before you start, here are few questions to ask yourself...

Q. Do you consider getting healthy a positive experience? If you're convinced making a healthy change will be a painful, negative experience, then that is likely what it will be. You create your own reality with your thoughts, so if your head is in a positive place about the change, the body is sure to follow.

Q. Are you ready to get moving? Trying to lose weight without physical activity is like trying to go scuba diving without oxygen. Getting active is an essential and necessary part of losing weight and keeping it off.

Q. Are you willing to learn from your "failures"? The road to a healthy life- style is fraught with challenges and you have to be willing to learn from your mistakes, as opposed to striving for unattainable perfection, and then quitting when the going gets tough.

Q. Are you ready to make a permanent change? Achieving and maintaining a healthy weight is a lifelong commitment that requires the implementation of permanent lifestyle solutions.

The Diet Thinker Challenge Overview
PART ONE: Gain Knowledge and Understanding
PART TWO: Collect and Decode Data
PART THREE: Design and Implement Your Weight Loss System

PART ONE: Gain Knowledge and Understanding
As you well know, information is power. The trouble is, with the endless supply of diet and health books on the market today and the influx of

conflicting and confusing nutrition information in the news, it can be time consuming and frustrating trying to separate weight loss fact from fiction. The tools and information provided in Chapter 7 (see page 203) cut through the confusion, providing the knowledge and understanding you need for success, and clearing up a few weight loss myths along the way. The first part of your challenge is to read Chapter 7 so you are well-equipped to make informed decisions about your health and well-being. While everything needed for ultimate success is provided in Chapter 7 for your Diet Type this abbreviated overview may not feel comprehensive. Not to worry—below is a list of scientific and trusted (optional) reading recommendations that you can research, review, and study to your Diet Thinker heart's content.

OPTIONAL READING RECOMMENDATIONS
YOU on a Diet by Michael Roizen and Mehmet Oz

This best-selling book from a trusted doctor team provides Diet Thinkers with their best weapon against weight gain: information. *YOU on a Diet* will show you how your brain, stomach, hormones, muscles, heart, genetics, and stress levels all interact biologically to determine how your body stores and burns fat.

Volumetrics Weight Control by Barbara Rolls and *The Volumetrics Eating Plan* by Barbara Rolls

Barbara Rolls, a respected food-nutrition researcher from Pennsylvania State University, explains "the science of satiety"—what researchers have learned about foods that make you feel full. You'll learn how to lose weight without feeling hungry by choosing foods that are low in calories, but high in volume.

The China Study by T. Colin Campbell

Called the "Grand Prix of epidemiology" by *The New York Times*, this study looks at more than 350 variables of health and nutrition with surveys from 6,500 adults in more than 2,500 counties across China and Taiwan. It conclusively shows the connection between nutrition and disease. The politics of health, food policy and nutrition as well as "the impact of special interest groups in the creation and dissemination of public information" are also reviewed.

What to Eat by Marion Nestle

This comprehensive review of the supermarket decodes, discusses and analyzes nutrition claims, labels and food shopping, and explores issues including the effects of food production on our environment, the politics of pricing, and the effect of additives on nutrition.

The Complete Idiots Guide to Total Nutrition by Joy Bauer

Don't let the name fool ya. This book is packed with useful info on everything from fats, cholesterol, carbohydrates, protein and supplements to exercise, food shopping, weight loss, and healthy eating.

The South Beach Diet by Arthur Agatston

If you are carb-sensitive (see page 207), a protein-lover, or are convinced that cutting the carbs is the way to go, be sure to do it in a nutritionally sound manner. *The South Beach Diet* is a reasonable choice. Agatston agrees with the entire medical community in believing that excess consumption of unhealthful "bad" fats contributes to an increase in cardiovascular disease, while the consumption of excessive carbohydrates contributes to obesity and diabetes. It is important to limit phase one of his diet to only two weeks as he recommends (even better, skip the phase altogether).

Remember that for a Diet Thinker weight loss often begins in the mind, and if you're not careful, it can end there. To keep yourself from getting caught in a never-ending cycle of research, designate yourself a specific amount of time (no more than two months) for your initial research. At the end of your allotted study time close your books, put your pencils down and move on to Part Two of your challenge. Moving on to Part Two certainly doesn't mean you have to stop learning or reading about nutrition and health, but it does mean you must take some action and put your valuable knowledge to good work. Of course, if you are a high achiever and want to start making changes in your life during Part One, please feel free, but later in your challenge you will be prompted to analyze your current health and habits (Part Two), and then to design and implement your weight loss system (Part Three).

PART TWO: Collect and Decode Data

While looking in the mirror or hoping on a scale is a good way to determine if you are overweight, it's particularly helpful for your Diet Type to take a closer look at your current health status and habits.

KNOW YOUR NUMBERS

BMI (Body Mass Index) is a measurement that describes the relationship between your height and your weight. It can be used to indicate if you are overweight, obese, underweight or at a healthy weight for your height.

Your BMI = ((Weight in Pounds) / (Height in inches)^2) x 703
(See page 232 for a BMI chart.)

18.5 or less	Underweight
18.5 to 24.99	Normal Weight
25 to 29.99	Overweight
30 to 34.99	Obese (class 1)
35 to 39.99	Obese (class 2)
40 or greater	Morbidly Obese

WAIST TO HIP RATIO

Waist-to-Hip ratio is a simple indication of your health status. To determine the ratio, divide your waist measurement by your hip measurement. For women, a ratio of 0.80 or less is considered safe, and a ratio of 1.0 or higher is considered 'at risk' for heart disease and other problems associated with being overweight. Grab a measuring tape, stand relaxed and no sucking in your gut! To find the circumference of your hips, measure at the widest part of your buttocks, and to find the circumference of your natural waist, measure just above the belly button.

BODY FAT PERCENTAGE

Your body fat percentage is the percentage of your weight which is made up of fat. It compares your body fat to your lean body mass, which is made up of bone, muscle and organ tissue. So, if your total body weight is 160 pounds and you have 32 pounds of fat, your body fat percentage is 20 percent.

Percent Body Fat for Women

Age	Good	Excellent
20-29	20.6-22.7	17.1-19.8
30-39	21.6-24.0	18.0-20.8
40-49	24.9-27.3	21.3-24.9
50-59	28.5-30.8	25.0-27.4
60-	29.3-31.8	25.1-28.5

The higher your percentage of fat is above acceptable levels, the higher your health risk for weight-related illness including heart disease, high blood pressure, and type 2 diabetes. Not to mention that because muscle is more metabolically active than fat, the higher your percentage of fat, the less calories you need to maintain your weight and the easier it is to pack on the pounds. There are several ways to determine your body fat percentage:

Hydrostatic Weighing: underwater weighing. This tried and true test is very accurate in determining percentage of body fat. Check your local university.

Skin-Fold Calipers: simple "pinch test" that measures the skin-fold thickness at several areas of your body. Accuracy depends on the tester. Check your local health clubs or university.

Bioelectrical Impedance (BIA): scales and hand-held devises that run low-level electrical current through your body; the faster the signal travels, the more muscle you have. Best results are obtained first thing in the morning with no alcohol consumed for 2 days prior, and no exercise the night before. This test can be obtained through local fitness centers, or check out amazon.com for some reasonably priced units you can use at home. There are even scales that will measure both your weight and do BIA.

VITAL STATS

If you've had a physical in the last 12 months call your doctor and obtain a record of your health data results including systolic and diastolic blood pressures, total cholesterol, LDL cholesterol, HDL cholesterol, triglycerides, and blood glucose and check them against acceptable levels. If you have not had a physical in the last 12 months, get one NOW.

Blood Pressure Levels

Classification of blood pressure for adults age 18 years and older

Category	Systolic (mm Hg)		Diastolic (mm Hg)
Normal	less than 120	And	less than 80
Prehypertension	120–139	Or	80–89
Hypertension			
Stage 1	140–159	Or	90–99
Stage 2	160 or higher	Or	100 or higher

Source: American Heart Association

Cholesterol Levels

Total Cholesterol Level	Category
Less than 200 mg/dL	Desirable level that puts you at lower risk for coronary heart disease. A cholesterol level of 200 mg/dL or higher raises your risk.
200 to 239 mg/dL	Borderline high
240 mg/dL and above	High blood cholesterol. A person with this level has more than twice the risk of coronary heart disease as someone whose cholesterol is below 200 mg/dL.

HDL Cholesterol Level	Category
Less than 40 mg/dL (for men) Less than 50 mg/dL (for women)	Low HDL cholesterol. A major risk factor for heart disease.
60 mg/dL and above	High HDL cholesterol. An HDL of 60 mg/dL and above is considered protective against heart disease.

LDL Cholesterol Level	Category
Less than 100 mg/dL	Optimal
100 to 129 mg/dL	Near or above optimal
130 to 159 mg/dL	Borderline high
160 to 189 mg/dL	High
190 mg/dL and above	Very high

Source: American Heart Association

TRIGLYCERIDE LEVELS

Category	Triglyceride Level
Normal	Less than 150 mg/dL
Borderline-high	150 to 199 mg/dL
High	200 to 499 mg/dL
Very high	500 mg/dL or higher
These are based on fasting plasma triglyceride levels.	

Source: American Heart Association

BLOOD GLUCOSE LEVELS

Levels up to 100 mg/dL are considered normal. Levels between 100 and 126 mg/dl are referred to as impaired fasting glucose or pre-diabetes and are considered to be risk factors for type 2 diabetes and its complications. Diabetes is typically diagnosed when fasting blood glucose levels are 126 mg/dl or higher.

Source: NIH

ANALYZE YOUR HABITS

It's time to put your analytical skills to good use by evaluating YOU. Now that you have properly informed yourself on the basics of healthy living you have the power to identify the possible health and weight loss downfalls in your own life.

Record your intake (food, time, and quantity), your physical activity, and your health habits for two weeks. Keeping a record will show the patterns that contribute to your health risks and assist you in developing a plan of action specific to your particular needs. Examine your patterns, evaluate your current diet and compare it against your nutritional needs, consider the big picture of your health and your life, and finally, brainstorm inventive solutions. Your time will be well invested as you can use the options you generate to help you design your weight loss system in Part Three of your challenge.

PART THREE: Design Your Weight Loss System

CALCULATE YOUR CALORIE NEEDS

The number of calories you take in and those you burn off determine weight loss, weight gain or weight maintenance. So, if you consume fewer calories than you burn, you will (duh) lose weight. You can do this by becoming more physically active, by eating less, or (preferably) by doing both. The first step is determining your calorie needs.

Your basal metabolic rate (BMR) is the rate at which your body burns calories while it's at rest.

Your BMR = 655 + (4.35 x weight in pounds) + (4.7 x height in inches) – (4.7 x age in years)

The Harris Benedict Equation uses your BMR and an activity factor to determine your total daily energy expenditure (calories). Multiply your BMR by the appropriate activity factor below to determine the approximate number of calories you need in order to maintain your current weight.

If you are sedentary (little or no exercise)
Multiply your BMR x 1.2

If you are lightly active (light exercise 1-3 days a week)
Multiply your BMR by 1.375

If you are moderately active (moderate exercise 3-5 days a week)
Multiply your BMR by 1.55

If you are very active (strenuous exercise 6-7 days a week)
Multiply your BMR by 1.725

If you are extremely active (very strenuous exercise everyday)
Multiply your BMR by 1.9

Once you know the number of calories you need to maintain your weight, you can calculate the number of calories you need in order to lose weight. You have to burn roughly 3,500 calories to lose a pound of fat, so to lose 1 pound a week you'll need to diet or exercise your way to a 500-calorie deficit each day. Keep in mind that the experts recommend that calorie levels never drop below 1,200 calories per day for women—and for active women this calorie level is considered quite low and may cause your metabolism to slow down. For active women I recommend an intake of around 1,600 calories per day.

STUDY DIFFERENT PLANS AND APPROACHES

Take a look at the weight loss plans and meal planning approaches in your optional reading recommendations as well as the information and meals in Chapter 8 (see page 239) and the structured approach for planning meals in the Diet Planner Plan on page 53 and the unstructured approach for picking meals in the Diet Player Strategy on page 92.

The meals in Chapter 8 make it easy for you to choose foods that deliver around 1,550 per day, with an optional 100 calories for Craving Tamers (Craving Tamers allow you to keep all your favorite foods in you life by simply slimming down the portions.) For most *active* females this will induce a healthy and safe weight loss of about two to three pounds a week. The meals in Chapter 8 are packed with all the nutrients you need for good health and weight loss, and you're also free to create your own meals using your own favorite foods and recipes using the guidance provided.

1,650 WEIGHT LOSS PLAN STATS

To provide adequate nutrients within calorie needs the 1,650 weight loss plan in Chapter 8. . .

- Has 20 to 30 percent of total calories from fat
- Has 40 to 60 percent of total calories from carbohydrates
- Has 15 to 40 percent of total calories from protein
- Has less than 10 percent of calories from saturated fat
- Has less than 300 mg of cholesterol
- Keeps trans fats and sugar as low as possible
- Provides around 1,000 mg of calcium
- Has no more than 2,300 mg of sodium
- Provides at least 25 g of fiber

BREAKDOWN FOR THE 1,650 CALORIE WEIGHT LOSS PLAN:

- 400 calorie breakfast
- 450 calorie lunch
- 550 calorie dinner
- 150 calorie snack
- 100 optional treat

NUTRITION PARAMETERS FOR THE 1,650 CALORIE WEIGHT LOSS PLAN:

Meal	Fiber, g At least	Sodium, mg Around	Sat Fat, g No more than	Calcium, mg Around
400 Breakfast	9	450	3	375
450 Lunch	8	600	4	125
550 Dinner	8	750	7	200
150 Snack	–	300	2	300
100 Optional Treat	–	200	–	–

BUILD AND IMPLEMENT YOUR WEIGHT LOSS SYSTEM

OK Diet Thinkers, it's time to take back control! Potent brain chemicals are in charge of giving us the signal to eat or not. Healthy eating is not a matter of willpower, it is a matter of feeding your brain and body what it needs so it doesn't falsely interpret the data you are inputting.

You can follow any of the recommended plans, one of the approaches in this book, or you can build your own healthy weight loss system based on all you have learned.

While beginning to implement your system be sure to set yourself up for success. This might include avoiding situations where you know you may be tempted. This could be avoiding office birthday parties where cake and candy are served, the break room where pastries are displayed in the morning, a co-workers cubical where they always have a bowl of candy, etc. This is a common practice in recovery programs such as AA, where newbies are encouraged to stay away from places where alcohol is being served. This recommendation is NOT forever, and should not be used as an excuse to avoid social functions! Typically it takes about 21 days to adopt a new behavior, and to allow your new patterns of behavior to integrate to the point that your identity will have shifted to a person that does not eat XYZ of food.

It's also not logical to keep tempting foods around that you know are going to throw you off track. While it is fine and appropriate to keep "Craving Tamers" around the house in small quantities, keeping big double sized bags of chips on the counter or gallons of ice cream in the freezer is not wise, and unnecessarily arouses temptation. It's suggested that you clear your house, office, and wherever, of tempting unhealthy foods.

PART THREE

Your Tools

CHAPTER 7

The Basics: The Truth and Nothing But the Truth!

In This Chapter...

Part One: You Really Are What You Eat

Calories Count

You count them, you cut them and you obsess about them, but have you ever considered just what a calorie is? Nutritionally speaking, a calorie is a measurement of energy from food.

Everything you eat, from a crunchy carrot stick to a slice of decadent cake, has calories. If you eat more calories than your body needs, you will gain weight. If you eat less, you will lose weight.

If you wanted to drop one pound, how much *less* would you have to eat? Well, one pound of body weight equals about 3,500 calories—so, to lose one pound, you would have to cut 3,500 calories from your diet over a period of time. If you dropped 500 calories a day, you would lose that weight in one week (500 calories x 7 days = 3,500 calories lost).

So if cutting calories equals weight loss, then *severely* cutting calories must mean super-fast weight loss, right? Wrong. When you suddenly and drastically reduce your calories, your body will assume you are in a state of emergency and automatically slow your metabolism so your system doesn't burn off its precious, "limited" supply of nourishment. A slow metabolism will make it extra hard for you to drop pounds—and that's not all. Even when you start eating normally again, your metabolism will remain sluggish for a time so that your "starving" body has a chance to regain weight as fast as possible. Yikes! Also, keep in mind that fast weight loss (more than two or three pounds a week), is mostly water loss, and losing water weight is not the same as losing fat. Losing water weight will leave you feeling dehydrated and drained, and you'll regain the water weight just as fast as you lost it. Plus, your insatiable hunger as a result of eating too few calories will set you up for a major diet setback, like a food binge.

A healthy diet (by the way, a "diet" is simply defined as what a person eats and drinks) shouldn't be miserable. Successful weight loss plans have enough calories to keep you from experiencing extreme hunger, but are also low enough in calories to allow for a moderate, safe weight loss of about two pounds per week.

To maintain overall health and provide your body with the nutrients it needs, as well as to keep your metabolism in check, a baseline level of around 1,200 calories per day is required. *However,* for active adult females, 1,200 is far too low. While exact calorie needs depend upon a variety of factors including height, weight and activity levels, for most women an intake of around 1,500 to 1,600 calories per day will lead to a healthy weight loss of about two pounds per week. You can maintain this calorie level for as long as it takes for you to reach your goals—be it weeks, months or even years.

The Balancing Act

Perhaps you've heard a friend say that she's cutting carbs (carbohydrates). Or maybe you've noticed a colleague only eating grapefruits in an effort to shimmy into a pair of jeans. Well, you may be surprised (and relieved!) to discover that such methods are *not* the best way to drop pounds. *The best weight loss plans incorporate all food groups and allow most foods in moderation.* Whether your calories come solely from grapefruit or from a well-balanced diet, as long as you keep the number of calories down, you will lose weight.

Want another reason to skip that grapefruit diet? Here it is: a well-rounded eating plan that contains all food groups will not only be much easier to stick to, but will also contain the variety of nutrients that your body needs to function at its peak. And when your body functions at an optimal level, you are more likely to feel satisfied, stay with the diet, and gain better results in the end.

Remember, once you take off the weight, you've got to maintain the loss. Yet another reason to commit to, a program that features a reasonable, well-rounded eating plan that teaches you how to eat well for life. Not to mention that eating right will help you feel, and look, your best!

Think of your body's needs in terms of a car. Everybody knows a car needs gas to run. A car needs oil too, but a lot of people don't think that's as important as gas. Skimp on the oil, though, and after a while your car will be sputtering and you'll have an expensive visit to the mechanic on your hands. The same type of thing happens to your body when you don't get a balance of nutrients in your diet. The calories you eat provide your body with what it needs to run (like gas in a car). However, a diet that lacks balanced nutrients will lead to health problems down the line, much like the effect of operating a car without oil. You might not feel the effects of an unbalanced diet right away, but the damage you do can be severe, and sometimes irreversible.

Basic human needs for survival, in terms of nutrition, are energy (calories), protein, carbohydrates, fat, vitamins, minerals and water. You get energy, vitamins and minerals from the macronutrients (aka: carbohydrates, protein and fat). While some foods are made up of mostly just one macronutrient (for example, pasta is mostly carbohydrate, chicken is mostly protein, and oil is fat), others (like a sandwich and lasagna) are a combo. Water comes from some foods, as well as whatever you add to your diet through water-based, decaffeinated beverages. By eating a balanced diet containing all of the macronutrients, you're giving your body the basic keys to survival that it needs to perform perfectly.

Breaking It Down: Be Choosy about Carbs

Carbohydrates. Carbs. Whatever you call them, most people think of them in much the same way: bread, pasta, cereal, grains and rice. But carbohydrates can be found in many other foods, including fruits, vegetables, sugars, and milk and other dairy products. While carbohydrates have gotten a bad rap in the world of weight loss, the truth is that they play a critical role in any diet because they are the main source of energy for all body functions and are necessary to metabolize other nutrients. Carbohydrates have four calories per gram—the same number of calories per gram as in protein. But all carbohydrates are not created equal.

There are two types of carbohydrates: simple and complex. Simple carbohydrates are broken down easily and quickly by the body to provide energy. Foods like cakes, candy, soft drinks—even milk products and fruit—are simple carbs. Complex carbohydrates have a more "complex" construction; thus, they don't break down as quickly to provide energy. Complex carbohydrates are foods like breads, rice and pasta.

When you're choosing carbohydrates to add to your diet, complex carbohydrates like whole grain pasta and bread, brown rice and legumes are the best to select since they are high in fiber (see Fiber: The Weight Loss Boss). Simple carbohydrates like low-fat dairy and fruit products are great choices, too, since they provide critical vitamins and minerals. However, steer clear of the sugary simple carbohydrates in candy, soda and cakes-they only take up space in your calorie budget, but provide nothing of substantial nutritional value. Approximately 40 to 60 percent of your total calories should come from carbohydrates.

～ FIBER: THE WEIGHT LOSS BOSS

Fiber is a type of carbohydrate that your body cannot digest; therefore it adds volume to fill you up without adding extra calories. Weight loss genius! A common complaint often expressed by people on a weight loss diet is, "I'm hungry." A wise dieter knows that it's not only how much you eat, but what you eat that makes the difference between a rumbling stomach and a full belly.

Fiber creates a sense of fullness that will leave you satisfied and better prepared to pass up seconds. If you build your meals and snacks around high fiber choices like whole grains, fruits and vegetables, and lean proteins and good fats, you'll have a great combination that will make it less likely you will overeat. In addition to helping you feel full, many (but not all) high fiber foods also have a lower glycemic index, meaning they don't cause your blood sugar to rise quickly after eating them. Without that rapid rise in blood sugar, you will likely eat less. Pitch refined carbohydrates like white bread and pasta in favor of whole grain choices, and you will experience the difference a bit of whole grain makes—you may even find that you prefer the nuttier more substantial taste and texture, too (see "How can you find the REAL whole grains hiding in your store?", page 208).

In addition to the weight loss benefits, studies show that a diet rich in fiber can help decrease your risk for colorectal cancer, heart disease and diabetes.

What If I Am Carbohydrate Sensitive?

A new term has emerged in recent years, along with the rise in diagnosed cases of diabetes: "carbohydrate sensitive." People who are carbohydrate-sensitive release more insulin than normal when they eat carbohydrates. This excess insulin increases storage of body fat and the risk of developing diabetes and heart disease. It also makes weight loss on a low-calorie, high-carb diet difficult and frustrating, because the insulin boost caused by high carbs inevitably leads to more fat.

Carb-modified plans (think *South Beach*, not *Atkins*) that focus on more protein from lean meat, fish, and low-fat dairy (about 40 percent of your total calories), "good" carbohydrates from whole grains and fruits and veggies (but less of them—also about 40 percent), and "good" polyunsaturated and monounsaturated fats (about 30 percent), offer an effective and healthy alternative to high-carb weight loss diets.

And a diet with moderate to low carbohydrates isn't just a good idea for those who are carb-sensitive. They can also work great for you if you like eating more protein, or if you have simply found that consuming fewer carbohydrates makes it easier for you to lose weight. Below, in Making the Best Choices (see page 214) and in Chapter 8, you'll find guidance on how to build healthy, delicious meals—whether you're a pasta-eating carb-lover or a carb-sensitive protein-lover. The "right" way is simply the way that works for *you*!

∼ HOW CAN YOU FIND THE **REAL** WHOLE GRAINS HIDING IN YOUR STORE?

Pick whole grains—that is grains that have not had their fiber-and nutrient-rich bran and germ removed by processing—over refined grains as often as possible. Look for bread, cereal, couscous, rice, crackers, pasta and other grain products that are 100% whole grain—meaning they contain NO refined flours. If the label does not say "100% whole grain," turn the package over and check out the ingredient list.

Whole grain ingredients to find: Whole Wheat, Oats, Rye, Brown rice, Bulgur wheat, Oatmeal, Barley, Buckwheat, Cracked wheat, Quinoa, Amaranth, Wild rice, Popcorn, Millet, and Spelt.

Refined ingredients to limit: Bleached or unbleached enriched wheat flour, White flour, Wheat flour, Semolina or durum flour, Rice flour, White rice, Cornmeal, and Corn flakes.

And don't be duped by products that claim to be an "excellent" or a "good source of" whole grain, or by label terms like "seven grain" "multi-grain," "whole grain blend," and "made with whole grain." These foods often contain far more refined grain than whole grain. Always check to see whether the predominant or first ingredient listed is a whole grain. The more fiber, the better. Also, keep in mind that all whole wheat products are whole grain since whole wheat is a type of whole grain, just like brown rice, oats, or bulgur.

∼ THE LOW-DOWN ON ARTIFICIAL SWEETENERS

While the safety of aspartame, acesulfame and saccharin is still questionable, Sucralose (aka Splenda)—sucrose (sugar) chemically combined with chlorine—has passed all safety tests, and is considered 100% safe. This is the sweetener that I use on a daily basis. Also keep in mind that there is nothing wrong with good-old fashioned sugar (white, brown, confectioner, or raw) or honey. The problem is that we tend to eat way too much of it. Limit yourself to around ten teaspoons of sugar (that's about 40 grams—be warned that a 12 ounce soda has around 39 grams of sugar) or less, per day.

Plenty of Powerful Protein

Proteins are made up of basic units called amino acids. Your body makes amino acids, but there are nine "essential" amino acids that you can only get from food.

Just as all carbohydrates aren't all the same, neither are proteins. Proteins are divided into two groups: complete and incomplete. Complete proteins have all nine essential amino acids. Examples of complete proteins are: meat, fish, poultry, eggs, milk products and soybeans. Incomplete proteins lack one or more of the nine essential amino acids—but they can still be great food choice. The best sources of incomplete proteins are: nuts, seeds, beans, peas and some grains.

Proteins are the major source of building material for muscles, blood, skin, hair, nails, and internal organs. Protein is also needed for the formation of hormones, enzymes, and antibodies, and for the proper elimination of waste material. Like carbohydrates, protein has four calories per gram, but where carbohydrates provide the body with fast-acting energy, protein provides long-term satiety and energy that lasts. When selecting protein from animal sources, be wary of fatty meats such as pork sausage and rib eye steaks. While they may be a source of protein, they can also be loaded with saturated fat, cholesterol and calories, not to mention nitrates, phosphates and other chemicals. Skinless chicken and turkey and fish are better everyday options. If you love red meat and pork, lean choices (like filet mignon, sirloin and London broil, pork loin, tenderloin, center loin and ham) are your better picks. About 15 to 40 percent of your total calories should come from protein. Remember, if you are carb-sensitive, your best bet is to stay on the high end of the protein range (40 percent).

～ VEGETARIANS AND PROTEIN

It was once thought that vegetarians needed to combine plant foods at every meal to ensure they consumed the right mix of proteins, but this idea is now defunct. Current research suggests that if you eat a variety of incomplete proteins within a 24-hour period (so that if one food is low in a particular essential amino acid, another food will make up this deficit) you will easily meet your protein and essential amino acid requirements.

~ DO YOU NEED TO BE CONCERNED ABOUT MERCURY CONTAMINATION IN FISH?

The Food and Drug Administration (FDA) and the Environmental Protection Agency advise women who may become pregnant, pregnant women, nursing mothers, and young children to avoid fish with high levels of mercury—such as shark, swordfish, king mackerel, or tilefish—and to limit any kind of fish to no more than two meals a week. The government also suggests this same group restrict canned albacore tuna to no more than 6 ounces per week, since canned albacore white tuna has three times more mercury than light. The rest of us don't need to be concerned. The latest FDA advisory says that up to 12 ounces of a variety of fish each week is safe for everyone. At 3 to 4 ounces per serving, the American Heart Association's target of 2 servings of fish per week is well below the FDA's safe limit. If you are concerned about picking eco-friendly seafood, check out these helpful websites for comprehensive and up-to-date information:

www.oceansalive.org

www.mbayaq.org/cr/seafoodwatch.asp

Fill Up with the Right Fats

Even when you're dieting to lose excess fat, you still need to include fat in your diet—just the right kind, and less of it. Like protein, fat helps you feel satisfied, and it also adds flavor to your food and serves many critical purposes in the body, acting as a fuel source for energy needs, and also providing insulation underneath the skin to maintain constant body temperature. Fat cushions vital organs against injury, and helps absorb vitamins A, E, D, and K. Of the macronutrients, fat, at nine calories per gram, weighs in as the most calorie-dense. It's for this reason that fat is included in a healthy diet, but with much more moderation than the other macronutrients. As you've been learning, all macronutrients have differences within each group, and fat is no exception.

Saturated and trans fat (see "What is trans fat?", page 211) are the primary culprits in raising dietary cholesterol, which increases the risk for coronary heart disease. Trans fat not only raises LDL (bad cholesterol), but can lower HDL (good cholesterol), too. You can find trans fat in fried foods like French fries, and in commercially baked products listing partially hydrogenated vegetable oil on the ingredient list. Saturated fat can be found in foods from animal sources like red meat, dairy, and a few plant-based sources like coconut and palm kernel oil.

Healthy fats include polyunsaturated and monounsaturated fats, two unsaturated fats that can help lower your LDL cholesterol and total cholesterol. Monounsaturated fat can help raise HDL, too. Instead of making saturated and trans fat-filled choices, substitute foods rich in monounsaturated or polyunsaturated fat like avocados, oils like olive, canola, corn, sunflower and soy oil, nuts, and Omega-3 fats derived from fish and flax. Around 20 to 30 percent of total caloric intake should come from fat.

~ IS MARGARINE BETTER THAN BUTTER?

Margarine is only better than butter if you use the right type. Some margarine brands are made with partially hydrogenated oil (PHO), which contain trans fat—which is as bad for your heart as the saturated fat found in butter. Choose trans-free spreads instead of margarines made with PHO. A warning: don't rely solely on the advertising on the front of a food package—check the nutrition label to be sure.

~ WHAT IS TRANS FAT?

While small amounts of trans fat occur naturally in meat and dairy products, that's not part of the trans fat issue you hear so much of these days. The big concern regarding trans fats is around manufactured food products. To keep foods fresh on the shelf or to turn liquid oils into solids (turning oil into margarine for instance), food manufacturers hydrogenate (add hydrogen to) polyunsaturated oils, creating unhealthy trans fat in the process. Thus, margarine, shortening, and cooking oils, as well as foods made with them, constitute a major source of unhealthy trans fat.

Be Wary of Liquid Traps

Alcohol isn't a macronutrient, but it does deliver a high dose of calories. At seven calories per gram, alcohol delivers more calories than protein and carbohydrates, but less than fat. Since alcohol has been shown to stimulate the appetite (and dull the senses) and often keeps high-calorie company with sugary mixers and calorie-laden bar snacks, it's easy to take in a lot of calories with a couple of drinks and a few handfuls of munchies. When you're watching your weight, keep in mind that for a couple hundred calories (maybe more, depending on your drink), you're not getting much nutrition. Whether you're dieting or not, alcohol is always best consumed in moderation, with women sticking to one drink per day. Choices like light beer and wine are better lower calorie options than cocktails that can be brimming in calories. One large frozen drink can easily contain as many (or more) calories as an entire meal!

And it's not just alcoholic drinks to keep your eye on. Drinks of any kind are an easy way to load your diet with extra calories. Sodas, fancy coffee drinks—even healthy drinks in excess like juice and milk—can spell trouble for your caloric bottom line if you drink too much. If you're thirsty, it's easy to gulp down hundreds of calories in juice before you even put down the cup. In general, try to leave the calories to food, with the exception of nutrient-dense drinks like milk. Even 100% juice isn't the best choice; eating the fruit itself is preferable to drinking it, since it ensures that you benefit from the fiber, too.

If you're looking for a thirst quencher that won't throw off your weight loss efforts but will still leave you satisfied, try a squeeze of lemon, grapefruit or lime in your water. For a change, plain unsweetened seltzer water is a great, calorie-free option, as are drinks like Hint and low-calorie Honest Tea. Coffee and tea are freebies too (just don't go overboard on the caffeine, cream and sugar).

THINK BEFORE YOU DRINK

Beverage (size)	Calories
Diet Coke or Diet Pepsi (20 oz.)	0
Water or club soda	0
Coffee, with one liquid creamer (8 oz.)	20
Tea, with two sugar packets (8 oz.)	20
Coffee, with one liquid creamer and one sugar packet (8 oz.)	30

Ocean Spray Light Cranberry Juice Cocktail *(8 oz.)*	40
Tropicana or Minute Maid Light Orange Juice *(8 oz.)*	50
V8 or tomato juice *(8 oz.)*	50
Dunkin' Donuts Coffee, with skim milk and sugar *(10 oz.)*	70
Silk Light Soymilk, Plain *(8 oz.)*	70
Milk, fat free *(8 oz.)*	80
Silk Light Soymilk, Vanilla *(8 oz.)*	80
Starbucks Cappuccino with skim milk, Grande *(16 oz.)*	80
Beer, light *(12 oz.)*	100
Milk, 1% *(8 oz.)*	100
Silk Soymilk, Plain or Vanilla *(8 oz.)*	100
Orange juice *(8 oz.)*	110
Red Bull *(8.3 oz.)*	110
Apple juice *(8 oz.)*	120
Dunkin' Donuts Coffee, with cream and sugar *(10 oz.)*	120
Milk, 2% *(8 oz.)*	120
Silk Light Soymilk, Chocolate *(8 oz.)*	120
Wine, white *(6 oz.)*	120
Starbucks Coffee Frappuccino Light, Grande *(16 oz.)*	130
Gatorade *(20 oz.)*	130
Glaceau Vitamin Water *(20 oz.)*	130
Starbucks Caffè Latte with skim milk, Grande *(16 oz.)*	130
Wine, red *(5 oz.)*	130
Cranberry juice cocktail *(8 oz.)*	140
Silk Chocolate Soymilk *(8 oz.)*	140
Grape juice *(8 oz.)*	150
Milk, whole *(8 oz.)*	150
Beer, regular *(12 oz.)*	160
Nestea Sweetened Lemon Iced Tea *(16 oz.)*	160
Gin and tonic, on the rocks *(7 oz.)*	190
Ginger ale *(20 oz.)*	200
Starbucks Cappuccino with whole milk, Venti *(20 oz.)*	210
Slim-Fast, canned *(11 oz.)*	220
Snapple Lemonade *(16 oz.)*	220
Starbucks Coffee Frappuccino, Grande *(16 oz.)*	240
Coca-Cola or 7-Up *(20 oz.)*	250
POM Wonderful 100% Pomegranate Juice *(16 oz.)*	320
Starbucks Caffè Latte with whole milk, Venti *(20 oz.)*	340
Starbucks Coffee Frappuccino, Venti *(24 oz.)*	350

Nestlè Nesquik Chocolate Milk *(16 oz)*	400
7-Eleven Super Big Gulp, Coca-Cola *(44 oz.)*	410
McDonald's Chocolate Triple Thick Shake, small *(16 oz.)*	580
Burger King Vanilla Shake, large *(32 oz.)*	820
Pina Colada *(16 oz.)*	880
Daiquiri *(16 oz.)*	900
McDonald's Chocolate Triple Thick Shake, large *(32 oz.)*	1,160
Smoothie King Chocolate or Strawberry Hulk *(32 oz.)*	1,530

Source: Manufacturers and U.S. Department of Agriculture.

~ THE DEAL WITH DAIRY

Fat free and 1% milk are lower in calories and saturated fat than their whole fat or 2% cousins. Same goes for low fat cheese, yogurt and other dairy products. However, the recommendations in this book are not for a low fat or fat free diet (see page 210, Fill Up with the Right Fats). Fat not only adds flavor to your meal and helps you feel satisfied, it is also needed for many, many critical bodily functions. The meals here provide a healthy and satisfying 20—30 percent of your calories from fat. And most of these fat calories come from heart-healthy unsaturated sources including olive and canola oils, nuts, and avocado. Also, if you're lactose intolerant, calcium-fortified soy milk, yogurt and cheese make excellent substitutions for dairy foods.

Making the Best Choices: Go for Nutrient Dense Deals

Think about it: if you're economizing on calories to lose weight, doesn't it make the most sense to pack a lot of nutrition into what you eat? Compare the concept of nutrient dense foods to shopping: for most people, a good shopping day is one where you're able to buy a high value product for a low price. It's the same with nutrition; a food that's value-packed with nutrients like vitamins and minerals, but isn't going to cost you a lot of calories is a nutritional bargain—it's a *nutrient dense* food. On the other hand, foods like candy, soda and sweets will set you back several hundred calories, but are low in vitamins and minerals, making them a low nutrient, or *calorie dense* food. Foods like these are also often called "empty calories"—empty of nutrients, that is! (see page 144 for an "Empty Calorie Overhaul"). By selecting empty-calorie foods, you're spending a lot of calories for something that offers nothing (like the insanely expensive, very cute shoes that give you blisters and are difficult to walk in. They might be OK to wear on occasion, but most of the time you'll want to wear cute *and* comfortable kicks.)

So how do you fill your diet with foods that are like that perfect pair of shoes, both fun *and* practical? Keep your diet simple and focus on balance and portions. It's as easy as 1, 2, 3 (OK, and 4!)...

Pick your Protein Your meal should always include some lean protein. If you're carb-sensitive (see page 207) or a protein-lover, have a little more protein (2 portions). If you're a carb-lover, simply have a little less (1 portion).

Pile on Produce Most of your meal should consist of nature's finest. Packed with nutrients and low in calories, nothing says healthy (and weight loss!) like veggies and fruits. There's no such thing as a bad fruit or veggie, but the more variety, the better. Stick with about two portions at your morning meal and have more (around three portions) for dinner and lunch. And try to pick veggies over fruit most of the time.

Grab your Grains Whole grains also deserve some space in your meal. Select fiber-rich, whole grain foods like oatmeal, whole wheat bread, and whole grain cereal, instead of refined grains like white bread, white pasta, and white rice. If you're a carb-lover have a little more whole grain (2 portions) and if you're a protein-lover, a little less (1 portion).

Finish with Fat A little fat goes a long, long way. Some olive oil in your salad, a little butter on your veggies, a handful of nuts with your cereal, or some avocado on your sandwich, all add satiety and flavor. Just one or two portions of fat makes a great meal!

To create a balanced 400-calorie breakfast simply Pick your Protein (1 portion for carb-lovers, 2 portions for protein-lovers), Pile on Produce (2 portions), Grab Your Grain (2 portions for carb lovers, 1 portion for protein-lovers), and Finish with Fat (1 portion). (See page 216 for portion information).

·   **To make a balanced 450-calorie lunch,** simply Pick your Protein (1 portion for carb-lovers, 2 portions for protein-lovers), Pile on Produce (3 portions), Grab Your Grain (2 portions for carb lovers, 1 portion for protein-lovers), and Finish with Fat (1 portion). (See portion information below).

For a balanced dinner of around 550 calories, simply Pick your Protein (1 portion for carb-lovers, 2 portions for protein-lovers), Pile on Produce (3 portions), Grab Your Grain (2 portions for carb lovers, 1 portion for protein-lovers), and Finish with Fat (2 portions). (See portion info in grey box below.)

Follow this easy meal-building guidance for breakfast (400 calories), lunch (450 calories) and dinner (550 calories), and stick with a calcium-rich snack (150 calories), and you'll get around 1,550 weight-reducing calories each day, plus all the nutrients you need for good health. You'll feel better, look better, and you'll drop pounds! See Chapter 8 on page 239 for some suggested meals.

Protein Portions

3 ounces of cooked lean meat, pork, fish, shellfish or skinless poultry
Turkey burger or veggie burger
2 eggs
4 egg whites
1 cup cooked beans
6 ounces of tofu
1 cup of low fat milk (or soy milk) or yogurt (or soy yogurt)
¾ cup low fat cottage cheese
2-ounces low fat cheese
½ cup low fat ricotta cheese

(Note: If you choose full-fat dairy products, choose smaller potions (about half) and cut back on your fat portions below.)

Produce Portions

2 cup of mixed greens or lettuce
1 cup raw veggies
½ cup cooked veggies
1 cup of berries or chopped fruit
½ cup grapes
1 piece of medium fruit
¼ cup dried fruit

Grain Portions

1 slice of whole grain bread
½ whole grain English muffin or whole grain bagel
½ cup cooked oatmeal
1 cup of cold whole grain cereal
½ cup whole grain pasta
½ cup whole wheat couscous, barley, quinoa, or other whole grain
1 medium whole grain roll
1 medium whole grain tortilla or pita
1 whole grain waffle
1 ounce whole wheat crackers (3 -5 crackers)
1 small baked potato or sweet potato (because these veggies are so starchy, they count as a grain serving)

Fat Portions

1 tsp oil, butter, trans-fee margarine, or mayo
2 tbsp reduced fat mayo or cream cheese
1 tbsp nuts or seeds
1 tbsp cream cheese, peanut butter or salad dressing
¼ small avocado
2 tbsp sour cream

Be Careful of Portion Distortion

While the above servings look great on paper, in the real world it's a little harder to estimate exactly what you're getting or just what counts as serving. When you're concentrating on losing weight, portion control is where the rubber really meets the road, so use these suggestions as a guideline to help you avoid portion distortion:

- ¼ cup (C)—one large egg
- ½ C—1 handful
- 1 C—the size of a tennis ball
- 1 oz. chicken, poultry, or meat—size of a matchbook
- 3 oz. cooked fish, poultry, or meat—size of a deck of cards
- 1 medium piece of fruit—size of a baseball
- 1 medium bagel—size of a hockey puck
- 1 oz. cheese—size of four dice

- 2 oz. cheese—size of a pair of dominos
- 1 small baked potato—size of a computer mouse
- 1 C raw vegetables, yogurt, or sliced fruit—as much as would fit into an average woman's hand.

All Foods Fit

So what about chips, doughnuts, crème brulee, milk shakes, my personal favorite bacon, and other, let's just say less-stellar choices? No food or drink (that's right NO food or drink) is so high in calories, fat or sugar that including them on occasion within overall healthful eating habits is going to cause problems. The key is making sure they are a small part of your overall diet. This might mean eating them only once in while, eating them in smaller portions, or eating less before of after your higher-calorie choices. It also helps to kick your activity into high gear so you can burn off those extra unwanted calories (see You Gotta Move It to Lose It page 223).

So if you have eggs Benedict and a side of bacon for breakfast every now and again (. . . uh, guilty), make up for it by watching your choices the next few days and putting in some extra time in at the gym. If you have six-course dinner including a cheese plate and a to-die-for chocolate turnover dessert once in a while (guilty), don't finish every bite of every course (you'll be uncomfortably full and unable to really enjoy the last few courses if you do) and spend the next few days being extra careful about your food and activity picks. And if you spend an August in Morocco drinking the Moroccan must-have thirst quencher—AKA orange Fanta (umm, guilty again), watch your other food and drink choices during the trip and when ya get home revert back to your normal, healthier drinking habits.

Some people like to plan indulgences, while others just go with the flow, either way you have learn to balance your choices and find a lifestyle that works for you (Diet Planners see page 25, Diet Players page 59, Diet Feelers page 99, and Diet Thinkers page 159). Sure, some indulgences balanced with more activity and better choices might result in weight maintenance instead of weight loss, but that's a heck of a lot better than weight gain. And in the overall picture of your weight loss efforts, weight maintenance some days, combined with weight loss most days, combined with a life you can enjoy is the way to go. This is not brain surgery; it's common sense.

Call me a disgrace to my profession but I am not willing to live a life that doesn't involve indulgence... and you don't have to either! Even if you are carefully watching calories you don't need to deprive yourself... not ever. (See Craving Tamers, page 262.)

A Multi a Day...

While hands-down, food, not pills, is the best way to get what your body needs, taking a multivitamin-and-mineral supplement is a sensible insurance policy to help you fill in the nutrition gaps. Look for a pill that has 100 percent of the Daily Value (often written as %DV—this is the Food and Drug's Administration's advice on how much of each vitamin and mineral to shoot for each day) for *most* vitamins and minerals. Taking this amount in a daily multi won't put you at risk of overdoing it, since the danger of dietary deficiencies is far greater than the risk of overdosing on vitamin and mineral supplements. Here's what you should look for in a multi...

Vitamin A:	no more than 4,000 IU
Beta Carotene:	no more than 5,000 IU
Vitamin C:	60-1,000 mg
Vitamin D:	at least 400 IU
Vitamin E:	30-100 IU
Vitamin K:	at least 20 mcg
Thiamin (B-1)	at least 1.2 mcg
Riboflavin (B-2)	at least 1.7 mcg
Niacin (B-3)	16-35 mg
Vitamin B-6	2-100 mcg
Folic Acid	no more than 400 mcg
Vitamin B-12	at least 6 mcg
Calcium	200 mg (if you are 51 or over you'll need to take a calcium supplement with 200-500 mg of calcium in addition to your multi.)
Iron	premenopausal 18 mg/ postmenopausal not more than 10 mg
Phosphorus	no more than 35 mg
Magnesium	100-350 mg
Zinc	8-23 mg
Copper	0.9-10 mg
Selenium	20-105 mcg
Chromium	at least 35 mcg

Unfortunately, dietary supplements aren't required to undergo the same testing as medicines, so picking a multi you can trust is tricky. Your best bet is to choose well-known mainstream brands and to also buy from large, trusted retailers. Also look on the bottle for a stamp from USP, NSF or ConsumerLab.com. While the stamp does not guarantee the product is safe and effective, it does show that the manufacturer has submitted the product for testing to show that it contains what is stated on the label.

MAKING THE OK DIET EVEN BETTER

Breakfast			
OK	**Better**	**Best**	**Why**
Large flavored bagel with regular cream cheese	Large egg bagel with fruit spread or low-fat cream cheese	Small whole-wheat bagel with peanut butter	A whole-wheat bagel has more fiber than either a flavored or an egg bagel, and peanut butter contains some protein and fat to keep you full longer.
Apple juice	Orange juice	One fresh orange	Apple juice is pretty much devoid of vitamins. Orange juice has more vitamins than apple juice, but a fresh orange contains fiber that the juice doesn't.
Sugary cold breakfast cereal with 2% milk	Instant oatmeal packet with skim milk	Old-fashioned rolled oats, cooked with raisins and diced apple, with a splash of calcium-fortified soy milk	The rolled oats contain more fiber than either the cold cereal or the instant oatmeal. The fruit and soy milk add a nutritional punch to the dish.
Pop-Tart®	Cereal bar with fruit filling	Nutritional/protein bar containing less than 200 calories and 5 grams of fat	The nutritional/protein bar contains less sugar, more protein, and more vitamins and minerals than either of the other choices.
Danish	Blueberry muffin	Oat bran muffin	The Danish and blueberry muffin both have more sugar and fat than the oat-bran muffin and also contain less fiber.

Lunch and Dinner			
OK	**Better**	**Best**	**Why**
Frozen French fries	Baked potato topped with margarine or light sour cream	Baked sweet potato fries	The frozen French fries are full of preservatives, sodium, and fat. Baked sweet potato fries have more vitamin A than the baked potato.
Cheeseburger with mayonnaise on bun	Lean turkey burger with mayonnaise and tomato on bun	Veggie burger with lettuce, tomato, onion, and mustard on whole-wheat bun	The veggie burger has more fiber, vitamins, antioxidants, and fiber than the other choices.
Italian hoagie	Ham and cheddar on white bread	Turkey breast and mozzarella on whole grain bread	The Italian hoagie has the most fat and sodium. The turkey breast sandwich has the least fat and the most fiber.
Cream of potato soup	Chicken noodle soup	Minestrone	Any cream-based soup is high in fat and cholesterol. Minestrone has more protein, fiber, and vitamins than chicken noodle soup.
Pepperoni pizza with cheese-stuffed crust	Plain cheese pizza on regular crust	Pizza with olives, onions, and peppers on thin crust	The pepperoni pizza with cheese-stuffed crust is high in fat, especially saturated fat and sodium. The plain cheese pizza would be a better choice. However, choosing a thin crust slashes the caloric and fat content of the slice, and the vegetables add vitamins, antioxidants, minerals, and a little fiber.
SpaghettiOs®	Pasta and sauce	Whole-Wheat pasta tossed with fresh vegetables and marinara sauce	SpaghettiOs® are full of preservatives and sodium. The whole-wheat pasta dish contains more fiber, vitamins, minerals, and antioxidants than plain pasta with sauce.

Snacks			
OK	**Better**	**Best**	**Why**
Fruit snacks	Fruit leather	Dried fruit	Dried fruit contains less sugar than either of the other choices.
Chocolate-chip cookie	Reduced-fat Devil's food cookie	Square of dark chocolate	While a square of dark chocolate does contain more fat than the devil's food cookie, it also boasts an impressive antioxidant level and will likely satiate your hunger better than either cookie.
Ice cream	Frozen yogurt	Fruit sorbet	Fruit sorbet contains less fat than either ice cream or frozen yogurt, and contains more vitamins and antioxidants because it is made from real fruit.
Potato chips	Pretzels	Baked tortilla chips with salsa	The pretzels and baked chips are both lower in fat than the potato chips, but the salsa can be counted toward your daily quota of fruits and vegetables.
Apple dumpling with vanilla ice cream and caramel sauce	Apple crumble	Baked apple stuffed with raisins and cinnamon	The apple dumpling contains much more fat than either of the other choices, and the baked apple contains much less sugar than the dumpling or the crumble.
Snack crackers with spinach or artichoke-and-cheese dip	Snack crackers with low-fat ranch dip	Whole Grain crackers with hummus	Spinach or artichoke dips do contain vegetables, but are also generally very high in fat, especially saturated fat. The whole grain crackers with hummus contain a healthier kind of fat, more fiber, more protein, and more vitamins and minerals than either of the other two choices.

Source: www.RD411.com

~ UNDER PRESSURE: SODIUM'S EFFECT ON YOUR HEALTH

If you are what you eat, then you are what you shake... salt, that is. Most people know that with a few flicks of the salt shaker, you can add additional and unnecessary sodium to your food. However, the salt shaker isn't the main culprit for the high amounts of sodium in the American diet. Restaurant meals and processed items can pack thousands of milligrams of sodium on their own. Considering that most healthy people should keep sodium intake below 2,400 milligrams per day, it's dangerously easy to overload on sodium with just a microwaved dinner and a run through the local drive through. Foods like lunch meats, canned soups, frozen meals, condiments, shelf-stable convenience meals, crackers, and instant cereals are the main sodium shamers.

Besides bringing on unsightly puffiness, what damage does a diet high in sodium do? Too much sodium in the diet increases your risk for high blood pressure, which can lead to heart and kidney disease as well as stroke. Though high sodium consumption isn't the only risk factor for these diseases, shaking sodium is one of the easiest to ways to stack the cards for good health in your favor.

It's not difficult to slash your sodium consumption. You can make big improvements simply by choosing to eat more freshly prepared foods, using lower sodium products, and removing the salt shaker from the table. Also, you'll have better control over your sodium intake if you limit the frequency in which you eat away from home.

Part Two: Ya Gotta Move It to Lose It

Exercise: Make it a Priority

Ginger and Fred, peanut butter and jelly, Romeo and Juliet: these are all pairs that are better together. The same goes for diet and exercise—both are good parts that, together, make an even better pair. Multiple studies on various population segments all indicate that weight loss results are much, much more effective with a combination of decreased calories and increased physical activity *together* than with either action independently.

If you follow a weight loss diet without exercise, you *will* be losing... but not just fat. You'll be losing critical lean muscle mass, too. Without exercise, diet alone results in the loss of ¼ lean body mass, and ¾ fat. A combination of reduced calories with increased physical activity can culminate in a loss of 98 percent body fat—much more efficient, since it's the fat, not lean tissue, that jiggles and wiggles. And because lean tissue requires more energy to run than fat, without exercise, you'd also be getting rid of an efficient fat burner—your own muscles! That's just plain counterproductive.

So how does exercise help you accomplish your weight loss goals? As you age, your Basal Metabolic Rate (BMR), or the number of calories your body uses while at rest, naturally slows. Increasing physical activity and building lean muscle mass can give your BMR a boost. After a vigorous work out, your BMR can remain increased for up to 48 hours for some people, meaning that even while you're taking a bubble bath, you're burning more calories than you would have if you hadn't exercised! Moderate physical activity actually suppresses appetite. Add to that the fact that, after you've sweated through a tough work out, you'll probably be a little less likely to give into a tempting candy bar that might undo all your good work, and there's no denying that exercise is one of your weight loss best friends.

Big Benefits

Need a few more reasons to lace up your sneakers? If you make an effort to exercise regularly, the benefits will go far beyond your initial goal of shedding pounds. To start, finding regular, enjoyable physical activity can boost your mood, build confidence, and relieve stress. You can even improve the quality of your rest, since research studies indicate that regular exercise decreases the time it takes to fall asleep and promotes longer, higher-quality shuteye.

You can also add chronic disease prevention to the growing list of exercise benefits. A healthy diet combined with exercise can cut your risk for chronic disease, since it lowers risk of type 2 diabetes and colorectal cancer. You've also probably heard that exercise is good for your heart—but exactly how good, you may wonder? Regular physical activity helps lower blood pressure, increases your good cholesterol (HDL) and decreases bad cholesterol (LDL), all working to lower your risk for heart disease. You can even feel the benefits of exercise right down to your bones, because weight bearing activities, like walking, dancing or aerobics helps prevent osteoporosis by building bone density. Need more encouragement to get moving? You can count on regular exercise to build flexibility, stamina and balance, helping to make everyday chores just a little easier.

How Much and What Type?

The amount of time you spend exercising, the rate of exertion, and your body weight all affect the amount of calories you burn while working out. The American College of Sports Medicine recommends 20-60 minutes of moderate aerobic exercise, 3-5 times a week. And if you include strength training (lifting weights) in your routine at least twice a week, you will build even more muscle and burn even more calories (and remember, your new muscles will keep bruning those calories even when you sleep!) Of course, the more you work out, the more you burn... and the more you burn, the more you can eat!

Aerobic exercise is any kind of exercise that gets your heart pumping. Lots of different types of activities can provide an aerobic work out. Biking, running, skiing, jumping rope, rollerblading, walking briskly and dancing all do the trick, as do stationary exercise machines like treadmills, stairsteppers and rowing machines. You can join a gym, go outside and run, ride a bike, or put in an exercise video at home. It's not what you do, or where you do it that really counts—as long as you *get moving*! If you've been inactive for a while, build up your activity *gradually*, starting at wherever you feel comfortable. Of course, before you start any new exercise program, it's wise to get your doctor's approval.

Also keep in mind that lifestyle activities such as gardening, yard work, washing your car, taking the stairs, and parking farther away from the store so you have further to walk are also helpful. That's because any time you increase activity, you burn calories. Take every chance you get to increase your daily activity and you'll see a big difference in your weight loss efforts.

BURN BABY BURN!

Some physical activities burn more calories than others. Below are the average number of calories a 154-pound person will burn, per hour, for a variety of activities. (A lighter person will burn fewer calories; a heavier person will burn more.)

Moderate Activity	Calories Burned
Hiking	370
Light gardening/yard work	330
Dancing	330
Golf (walking and carrying clubs)	330
Bicycling (less than 10 mph)	290
Walking (3.5 mph)	280
Weight lifting (light work out)	220
Stretching	180

Moderate Physical Activity Calories Burned per Hour

Vigorous Activity	Calories Burned
Running/jogging	590
Bicycling (more than 10 mph)	590
Swimming (slow freestyle laps)	510
Aerobics	480
Walking (4.5 mph)	460
Heavy yard work	440
Weight lifting (vigorous work out)	440
Basketball (vigorous)	440

Vigorous Physical Activity Calories Burned per Hour

Source: Adapted from the 2005 Dietary Guidelines Advisory Committee Report

LOOKING TO HIRE A PERSONAL TRAINER? CONSIDER THIS...

The Diet Planner requires an experienced, dependable, committed trainer—one that is on-time and professional. They want someone that will help them set clear goals, define specific steps for achieving these goals, and provide the details necessary to perform their exercise work outs effectively. Diet Planners like to follow plans that are "tried and true," "doctor recommended," and "time tested." Trainers that promote new-fangled fads hold little appeal to a Diet Planner, who expects consistency, reliability and tangible measurements of her progress. A little recognition goes a long way for Diet Planners, whose secret dream-come-true just might be receiving a "Certificate of Successful Completion."

The Diet Player is attracted to power, style and sexiness in a trainer. They want someone they can drool over and possibly impress at the same time. Diet Players love to be pushed to their limits and might even find it helpful when a trainer shouts commands during a work out. If they can flirt, it increases the fun. Diet Players want variety in their work outs and don't mind working up a sweat or being teased into action. A little competition, either with themselves or against someone else,some loud, motivating music, and an action-packed environment helps to keep a Diet Player engaged.

The Diet Feeler is drawn to trainers that are compassionate, empathetic, and non-judgmental. They want someone to inspire them, so they would really appreciate a trainer that has previously struggled with their own weight or exercise challenges. Diet Feelers want to be able to converse and connect during a work out, and they like it when their trainer's energy level is on par with or slightly higher than their own. If a trainer's energy level greatly surpasses the Diet Feelers', they can perceive the trainer as "too intense," as well as "pushy" or "aggressive." Diet Feelers are most comfortable when their trainer is friendly, accepts them for who they are, and encourages them to go at their own pace.

The Diet Thinker seeks out credentialed professionals that have a background in nutrition and exercise science. The want someone who can answer their questions, and they want to be confident that the answers will be based on factual, well-researched information. If a Diet Thinker asks a question and the trainer does not know the answer, the Diet Thinker will expect that the trainer will provide her with a credible web resource so she can look it up herself. Because they have a keen sense of humor, Diet Thinkers also appreciate someone with wit.

Part Three: Debunking Diet Myths

In the diet-obsessed world we live in today, diet myths have run amok! Everyday a new diet, pill, or book promises to be the latest and greatest weight loss fad, only to lead to to frustration and eventual failure for thousands.

Diet myths not only thwart your weight loss goals; they can also be downright unhealthy. Here's what you need to know to separate weight loss fact from fiction.

Myth: Diet pills can help you lose weight.

Truth: There is no such thing as a quick-fix, magic pill when it comes to weight loss. Pills don't teach you to make long-term, healthy changes you can live with, and they don't build fat-burning muscle. Bottom line: save your money.

Myth: Food cravings indicate your body needs something.

Truth: The reason we crave certain foods has never been scientifically proven. While some experts think it could have something to do with hormonal changes, most women just crave the foods they enjoy eating. Cravings can also be brought on by visual triggers (like seeing a juicy burger on a commercial), sensory triggers (like smelling freshly baked bread) or even emotional triggers (like anger or sadness).

Myth: Drastically cutting calories helps you lose weight.

Truth: Actually, when you don't eat enough calories, you send your body into starvation mode. The result? Your metabolism slows down so your "starving" body can maintain its weight. It goes without saying that a slow metabolism certainly doesn't help you when you are trying to lose weight! The trick is to reduce your calories enough to lose weight, but not so much that you negatively affect your metabolism or make yourself hungry. For most active females, a caloric intake of about 1,600 calories per day will induce a healthy weight loss of about two pounds per week.

Myth: Fat makes you fat.

Truth: Excess calories make you fat, and while fat has more calories per gram (9 calories) than carbs and protein (4 calories), if you pack an extra 2,000 calories a day into your diet it's not going to matter if those calories come from butter, pasta or chicken. The truth is, fat needs to be included in a healthy well-balanced diet, so, rather than eliminate it from your diet, you should choose the best types of fat and enjoy them in moderation. These "good fats" include monounsaturated or polyunsaturated fat found in foods like avocados, oils like olive, canola, corn, sunflower and soy oils, nuts, and Omega-3 fats derived from fish and flax.

Myth: Carbohydrates make you fat.

Truth: Again, it is extra calories that make you fat. It does not matter if those calories come from carbs, fat, protein or alcohol—if you take in too many calories, those calories will turn to fat. Instead of "cutting carbs," reduce your consumption of refined carbs and load up on whole grains, fruits and veggies instead.

Myth: Eating just one kind of food helps you shed pounds.

Truth: Whether you're talking about only eating grapefruit, cabbage soup or whatever they call for in the latest fad, the only reason you lose weight on this type of restrictive, one-food-only diet is because of a lack of calories. This type of restrictive eating can't be sustained in the long-term and they can lead to dangerous deficiencies. In short, these diets not only lack nutrients and variety—they also lack plain ol' common sense.

Myth: Eating protein and carbs at different meals will help you slim down.

Truth: The idea here is that because your body uses different enzymes to digest different types of foods, eating carbs (like a potato) and protein (such as a steak) separately will improve digestion and increase weight loss. Not true. Your digestive system is designed to handle lots of different foods at the same time and there is *zippo* scientific proof that eating certain foods individually will encourage weight loss.

Myth: You have to break a sweat while exercising in order to burn calories.

Truth: Any time that you increase activity, you burn calories. True, you burn more calories running on treadmill than just walking around the block, but you also burn more calories taking a walk than sitting on the couch. One of the easiest ways to burn more calories is to add more activity to your daily routine. For example, walk or ride your bike to work, take the dog on longer walks, always opt for the stairs, and park a few blocks away from your destination.

Myth: Body fat can be turned into muscle.

Truth: Fat and muscle are two different animals. You burn fat and you build muscle, but there is no mechanism that transforms fat into muscle. It's just not possible.

Myth: Fad diets work for long-term weight loss.

Truth: Fad diets, which usually promise speedy weight loss and insist you cut out certain foods or even entire food groups, are not long-term solutions. Not only are these un-balanced diets unhealthy, dieters regain any weight lost more often then not. That's because temporary changes don't equate to permanent losses. Research shows that a moderate weight loss of around 2 two pounds per week through healthy, varied food choices, physical activity, and permanent lifestyle solutions including portion control, is the best way to lose weight—and keep it off. That's because temporary changes don't equate to permanent losses.

Myth: Skipping meals helps you lose weight.

Truth: Many people think that when they skip meals, they eat less food, and therefore they lose more weight. But when you skip meals, your metabolism not only drops, you also tend to overeat at your next meal. So skipping meals may actually make you *gain* weight. Studies show that people who eat breakfast (the most commonly skipped meal) are more successful at weight loss than folks who ditch their morning meal.

Myth: Eating late at night will make you gain weight.

Truth: The time of day that you eat is not nearly as important as how much you eat and how much you burn. It doesn't matter if you eat your calories in the morning or at midnight; if you eat excess calories at *any* time they will turn to fat. However, all things considered, it's best to consume your calories during the day, since that's when your body needs the fuel.

Myth: Caffeine speeds up your metabolism and helps you drop pounds.

Truth: Caffeine can temporarily speed up your metabolism for a short time, but not enough to cause weight loss.

Myth: Foods labeled as "low" or "light" are always low in calories.

Truth: Often, these foods contain other flavor-enhancing ingredients that add calories. Some low-fat and fat-free foods even have as many calories as their full-fat versions. When you are watching your weight, the bottom line is calories, so be sure to flip that "diet" product over and investigate the numbers before you dig in.

Part Four: Ready, Set, GOAL!

The Scoop on BMI

If you've bought this book, it's likely that you have already pondered how much weight you want to lose. Maybe it's ten pounds; maybe it's 100. Regardless of how much you think you *need* to lose, before you begin, take the time to determine a healthy weight for you. One reliable source is the

Body Mass Index (BMI), which calculates an individual's body fat based on height and weight (see chart below). Based on where your results fall on the the BMI scale, a person may be classified as underweight, normal weight, overweight, or obese.

Like any calculated measurement, BMI does have limitations, but when used as a screening guide to gauge health risk related to weight, it is very effective. BMI is best used to determine a healthy weight for people ages 19-70, and shouldn't be used by women who are pregnant or nursing, competitive athletes, body builders, and chronically ill patients.

Here's the BMI breakdown:

18.5 or less	Underweight
18.5 to 24.99	Normal Weight
25 to 29.99	Overweight
30 to 34.99	Obese (class 1)
35 to 39.99	Obese (class 2)
40 or greater	Morbidly Obese

BODY WEIGHT IN POUNDS ACCORDING TO HEIGHT AND BODY MASS INDEX.

BMI	19	20	21	22	23	24	25	26	27	28	29	30	31	32	33	34	35
Height (inches)	Body Weight (pounds)																
58	91	96	100	105	110	115	119	124	129	134	138	143	148	153	158	162	167
59	94	99	104	109	114	119	124	128	133	138	143	148	153	158	163	168	173
60	97	102	107	112	118	123	128	133	138	143	148	153	158	163	168	174	179
61	100	106	111	116	122	127	132	137	143	148	153	158	164	169	174	180	185
62	104	109	115	120	126	131	136	142	147	153	158	164	169	175	180	186	191
63	107	113	118	124	130	135	141	146	152	158	163	169	175	180	186	191	197
64	110	116	122	128	134	140	145	151	157	163	169	174	180	186	192	197	204
65	114	120	126	132	138	144	150	156	162	168	174	180	186	192	198	204	210
66	118	124	130	136	142	148	155	161	167	173	179	186	192	198	204	210	216
67	121	127	134	140	146	153	159	166	172	178	185	191	198	204	211	217	223
68	125	131	138	144	151	158	164	171	177	184	190	197	203	210	216	223	230
69	128	135	142	149	155	162	169	176	182	189	196	203	209	216	223	230	236
70	132	139	146	153	160	167	174	181	188	195	202	209	216	222	229	236	243
71	136	143	150	157	165	172	179	186	193	200	208	215	222	229	236	243	250
72	140	147	154	162	169	177	184	191	199	206	213	221	228	235	242	250	258
73	144	151	159	166	174	182	189	197	204	212	219	227	235	242	250	257	265
74	148	155	163	171	179	186	194	202	210	218	225	233	241	249	256	264	272
75	152	160	168	176	184	192	200	208	216	224	232	240	248	256	264	272	279
76	156	164	172	180	189	197	205	213	221	230	238	246	254	263	271	279	287

Take a look at the BMI chart to see where you fall on the scale based on your current weight and height. If your BMI is 25 or above, losing weight will be an important step to improve your health and reduce your risk of chronic diseases. People with a BMI of 25 or above are at greater risk for hypertension, high cholesterol, type 2 diabetes, coronary heart disease, stroke, gallbladder disease, osteoarthritis, sleep apnea and some types of cancer.

How to Use BMI to Reach Your Own Personal Goal

To get to your weight loss destination, it helps to know where you are heading. Before you start your weight loss plan, take a moment to determine your weight loss goal.

Start by establishing your long-term weight loss goal, or your target weight.

A healthy weight for you is one that falls within a BMI of 18.5–24.9. The good news is that you don't have to aim for a specific number, but rather a wide range.(for example, a person who is 5'5" tall is within a healthy weight range if they weigh between 114–144 pounds.) Once you have determined your BMI, you will know where you stand, and how many pounds you need to lose to place you within a healthy weight range. You can also base your target weight on a doctor's suggestion or a previous desirable weight. It's really up to you how much you want to lose, but you need to keep your target weight reasonable. And no, your weight if you were a super model or your weight after spending three months on a deserted island, are *not* realistic goals!

Once you have established your long-term target weight goal, you'll need to establish your short-term goal. Why? Well, while your target weight might seem a bit overwhelming at first, your short-term goal, or as I like to call it, your "in-between" weight (a mere 5 percent of your current weight), will seem completely attainable. *And it is!* Achieving your short-term goal will not only have a positive impact on your health, but also on your state of mind. This will enable you to get to your target weight, one manageable goal at a time.

So, if your starting weight is 160 pounds, your "in-between" weight is 152 pounds (you calculate 5 percent of 160 like this: 160 x .05 = 8; 160 − 8 = 152). Once you accomplish your short-term weight loss goal of 152 pounds, you simply set a new "in-between" goal-weight of 145.5 pounds.

(again, 5 percent of your current weight: 152 x .05 = 7.5, 152 – 7.5 = 144.5). You will repeat this pattern until you reach your target weight. Remember, you will be losing weight at a healthy rate of about two pounds per week, and you should guesstimate the time it will take you to reach your in-between weight based on that two pounds per week rate.

Also keep in mind that weekly (not daily!) weigh-ins provide a better gauge of where you are in the pounds department. Just be sure to weigh yourself at the same time (preferably in the morning), on the same day of the week, using the same scale. And for best results, try weighing yourself in the buff. Note that the scale is not the only way to measure progress: take body measurements with a tape measure, test your body fat percentage, compare personal photos over time, and assess the fit of your clothing to monitor your improvements. If you are a Diet Feeler or Diet Player, you may want to simply pull out your skinny jeans or the clothes in your closet that you would like to get back into and use them to gauge your progress. Planners and Thinkers usually fair well with a focus on the scale.

If you have a setback, don't throw in the towel! Getting to your goal means keeping focused, bending when you need to bend, and getting back into the game when you've had a wipeout.

Use the guidance from your Diet Type chapter and the meals in Chapter 8 to help you build your eating plan, create your healthy life and lose weight.

Diet Planners—see page 25
Diet Players—see page 59
Diet Feelers—see page 99
Diet Thinkers—see page 159

RESTAURANT RUNDOWN

Plenty of great meal options abound in eating establishments; from all-American diners to the most exotic edibles, there's always a good dish choice available for you. The tips below are just what you need to make the best choices when you are away from home.

- **Get Informed by Going Online**—Many restaurants post their entire menu plus nutrition information online, making it easy to make an informed choice.

- **Have a Snack**—With a snack in your stomach, you will be less likely to overindulge on the first thing that you see. Have a small, balanced snack containing a little protein, fat and fiber (like one slice of whole grain toast with a tablespoon of peanut butter) before you go out to eat.

- **Your Server, Your Friend**—Think of your server as your link to the kitchen; they can tell you how the food is prepared, suggest healthier substitutions, and be your advocate for special requests like "easy on the oil."

- **Clue in with Key Words**—The description on the menu can tell you a lot about how a food is prepared. Words like "fried," "battered," "crispy," "au gratin," "scalloped," and "creamed" usually mean big-time calories, plus trans or artery-clogging saturated fat. Instead, look for healthy key words like "grilled," "blackened," "baked," "broiled" (but not in butter!), or "dry roasted."

- **Ban the Buffet**—It is possible to make decent choices on the buffet, but the temptation to overindulge on fat and calories (and to feel you're getting your money's worth) can get you into diet trouble. The best solution is to stick to the regular menu, where the limitations on portions can save you hundreds of calories.

- **Be Wary of the "Diet Menu"**—In many cases, the diet menu isn't really "diet" at all. Look carefully at each choice on the diet menu, and keep an open mind about the rest of the menu—you may find the best choices are in the other sections.

- **Start with a Salad**—Whether your main dish will be pizza or pasta, steak or seafood, starting with a garden salad dressed with a low fat vinaigrette can fill you up with fiber and a healthy dose of antioxidants...and leaves you with less room for the higher calorie entrée.

- **Ask for a Low Fat Version**—Many restaurants have low fat versions of the regular thing (like mayo, sour cream, or milk). Ask if your restaurant has healthier choices—you may be pleasantly surprised!

- **Avoid Unnecessary Temptations**—If the tortilla chips or breadbasket that are automatically brought to your table sabotage your best intentions before the meal officially starts, simply ask your server to keep it in the kitchen.

- **Stick to Simple**—The more a dish is dressed up and added to, the more calories and fat it usually has. Take a specialty sandwich; what makes it special? Probably a creamy, fat-laden "signature sauce" topped with tangy cheese, sandwiched between slabs of buttery bread. A simple turkey sandwich with flavorful mustard on whole wheat is a much healthier choice (you can add avocado, a "friendly fat," or some low-fat cheese for your own version of a sandwich that is truly special—in more ways than one!).

- **You're the Boss**—Want the grilled chicken club, but don't need the bacon, cheese and mayo, as well as the accompanying fries? Order your meal "your way" by asking the server to hold off the things you don't want, or inquire about substitutions. Almost all restaurants will be more than happy to accommodate your requests.

- **Split it or Save it**—Many restaurant meals are gargantuan. If you notice the meal is bigger than you need (and it probably is) ask your server to bring you a takeout container to divide your meal before you dig in. You'll have another meal tomorrow! Better yet, split your meal with a dining companion.

- **Get Smart with à la Carte**—If you don't see an entrée on the menu that fits your specifications, build your own from the a la cart menu. Shrimp cocktail, salad, and a baked potato make a satisfying meal, and may not be grouped together on the menu—but are listed separately on the à la carte menu.

- **The Best Call is Always Small**—Aim to choose the smallest portions when you can: a petite cut steak, a small ice cream cone, a half of a sandwich. Diminutive meal portions can be supplemented with healthy extras like veggies, fruit, and broth-based soups, while small portions of desserts like ice cream can give you the flavor you crave without blowing your diet.

- **Put it on the Side**—Be sure you ask for sauces and dressings on the side, instead of having them added to your meal in the kitchen. You can control the amount you use, and enjoy the natural flavor of the foods without having them drowned in extra fat and calories.

- **You Don't Have to Desert Dessert**—If you want something sweet to wrap up your meal, ask your server about fresh fruit or sorbet. When something sinful is calling your name, share it with a couple of dining companions to distribute the caloric impact.

- **Expand your Knowledge**—There are many books available on the topic of healthy eating in restaurants. And, best of all, the more you read, the easier it will become for you to make smart choices when you're out. Books like *Restaurant Confidential*, by Michael Jacobson and Jayne Hurley or *Eat This, Not That*, by David Zinczenko are great titles to explore.

CHAPTER 8
The Meals

In This Chapter...
- 400-Calorie Breakfasts
- 450-Calorie Lunches
- 550-Calorie Dinners
- 150-Calorie Snacks
- 100-Calorie Craving Tamers

Using the guidance from your Diet Type chapter, use these meals to help you build your eating plan, create your healthy life and lose weight. Combine your picks with regular exercise (see page 223) and you'll drop pounds, feel satisfied, enjoy delicious foods, and train yourself to eat right and cook healthy—for life. *Note: for a complete breakdown on the nutrition parameters of these meals, please see page 198.*

Diet Planners—see page 25
Diet Players—see page 59
Diet Feelers—see page 99
Diet Thinkers—see page 159

These tasty and easy-to-prepare meals were created by Tamara Goldis (a Diet Feeler). The talented Tamara is not only a registered dietitian; she is also trained as a Chef with an A.A.S in Culinary Arts and a B.S. in Culinary Nutrition from Johnson & Wales University. Tamara started her career at Oxmoor House, the cookbook division of Southern Progress, where she tested and developed recipes for Weight Watchers, *Cooking Light* and *Southern Living*. Next she spent a few years working at CSPI creating recipes for the *Nutrition Action Healthletter*.

These meals use lots of fresh fruit and vegetables, lean proteins like chicken, turkey, and fish, high-fiber whole grains breads and cereals, and healthy fats like avocado, olive oil, and canola oil. Using whatever is seasonal and available, feel free to swap like foods—mango for banana, pecans for almonds, chicken for turkey, etc.—and to create your own meals using the guidance below. The possibilities of calorie-appropriate, delicious and tasty meals are limitless! My favorite go-to places to look for recipes on the web are www.myrecipes.com and www.epicurious.com. I'm also a long-time subscriber of *Cooking Light* and my favorite cookbooks include the *Eat, Shrink, and Be Merry* by Janet Podleski and Greta Podleski and *The Best Life Diet Cookbook* by Bob Greene.

The following meals are for one serving—that way you don't have to worry about trying to divide the ingredients if you're just cooking for yourself. But, if you'd like your whole family to have the same thing for dinner, or you're just cooking for you and a friend, it's fairly easy to double (or even triple and quadruple) the meals. Just double the amounts that are listed for each ingredient to make two servings (or more).

400-Calorie Breakfasts

Create Your Own Breakfast: While any recipe or combo of foods that provides around 400 calories will do the trick, to create a balanced 400-calorie breakfast simply Pick your Protein (1 portion for carb-lovers, 2 portions for protein-lovers), Pile on Produce (2 portions), Grab Your Grain (2 portions for carb lovers, 1 portion for protein-lovers), and Finish with Fat (1 portion). (See portion info on page 216.)

BASIL SCRAMBLE

Sauté ¼ cup each chopped portobello mushroom and red onion with 2 tbsp. chopped red pepper in a nonstick skillet coated with cooking spray until tender, about 4 minutes. Stir in 1 whole egg and 2 egg whites and scramble until cooked through, about 3 minutes. Season with ⅛ tsp. black pepper and 1 tsp. chopped fresh basil. Serve with 1 slice whole grain toast spread with 2 tsp. trans free margarine or light butter (such as Land O'Lakes Light Butter with Canola Oil), ¾ cup nonfat milk, and 1 cup berries.

Calories: 420
Protein: 26 g
Carbohydrate: 53 g
Fiber: 9 g
Total Fat: 13 g

Saturated Fat: 3 g
Cholesterol: 215 mg
Calcium: 400 mg
Sodium: 500 mg

Lower-Carb Option: Skip the toast and have 3 oz. lean turkey or chicken sausage, lean meat (such as Hormel Natural Choice), or veggie sausage (such as Morningstar Farms Veggie Sausage Patties).

CHOCOLATE RASPBERRY SMOOTHIE

In a blender, combine 1½ cups light chocolate soy milk (such as Silk Light) with 1 cup raspberries (fresh or frozen), ½ cup vanilla lowfat yogurt and ¼ tsp. cinnamon. Blend until smooth. Serve with 1 slice whole grain toast spread with 1 tsp. trans free margarine or light butter (such as Land O'Lakes Light Butter with Canola Oil) and 2 tsp. raspberry preserves.

Calories: 410
Protein: 20 g
Carbohydrate: 68 g
Fiber: 10 g
Total Fat: 8 g

Saturated Fat: 3 g
Cholesterol: 11 mg
Calcium: 700 mg
Sodium: 480 mg

Lower-Carb Option: Skip the toast and have 2 tbsp. mixed nuts.

RASPBERRY FRENCH TOAST

Whisk together 1 egg, ¼ cup nonfat milk, ½ tsp. cinnamon and 1 tsp. vanilla. Pour mixture over 2 slices whole grain bread. Sauté in a nonstick skillet coated with cooking spray 3–4 minutes on each side or until golden. Top with 1 tbsp. maple syrup, ½ cup fresh raspberries and 1 tbsp. chopped pecans. Serve with ½ cup lowfat yogurt.

Calories: 420
Protein: 22 g
Carbohydrate: 62 g
Fiber: 13 g
Total Fat: 14 g

Saturated Fat: 3 g
Cholesterol: 220 mg
Calcium: 470 mg
Sodium: 340 mg

Lower-Carb Option: Have just one piece of French toast and another tbsp. pecans.

YOGURT PARFAIT

Combine ½ cup high-fiber cereal (such as Kashi Heart to Heart) with 1 tbsp. slivered almonds, ¼ cup mixed dried fruit, and ¼ tsp. allspice. Top with ¾ cup plain lowfat yogurt (such as Fage Total 0% or Oikos Greek) mixed with 2 tsp. honey. Serve with a clementine.

Calories: 400
Protein: 16 g
Carbohydrate: 66 g
Fiber: 8 g
Total Fat: 12 g

Saturated Fat: 2 g
Cholesterol: 11 mg
Calcium: 391 mg
Sodium: 240 mg

Lower-Carb Option: Have just ¼ cup cereal and have 1 part skim cheese stick.

INSTANT OATMEAL BREAKFAST

Cook 1 package of instant oatmeal (such as Quaker Simple Harvest Maple Brown Sugar with Pecans) according to package directions. Stir in ¼ cup chopped apple, 2 tbsp. chopped dates, and 1 tbsp. pecans. Serve with ½ cup lowfat yogurt mixed with ¼ cup berries.

Calories: 400
Protein: 13 g
Carbohydrate: 63 g
Fiber: 9 g
Total Fat: 14 g

Saturated Fat: 1 g
Cholesterol: 5 mg
Calcium: 365 mg
Sodium: 310 mg

Lower-Carb Option: Skip this meal.

COLD CEREAL BREAKFAST

Combine 1 cup high-fiber cereal (such as Kashi Go Lean) with ⅓ cup blueberries and 1½ tbsp. almonds. Top with 1 cup nonfat milk. Serve with a clementine.

Calories: 390
Protein: 27 g
Carbohydrate: 54 g
Fiber: 14 g
Total Fat: 13 g

Saturated Fat: 1 g
Cholesterol: 5 mg
Calcium: 438 mg
Sodium: 260 mg

Lower-Carb Option: Have just ½ cup of cereal and ½ cup milk, and have 3 oz. lean turkey or chicken sausage, lean meat (such as Hormel Natural Choice), or veggie sausage (such as Morningstar Farms Veggie Sausage Patties).

PEACH BLACKBERRY SMOOTHIE

In a blender, combine 1 cup plain lowfat yogurt (such as Fage Total 0% or Oikos Greek) with 1 cup frozen peaches, ¼ cup blackberries (fresh or frozen) and 1 tbsp. maple syrup. Serve with 1 slice whole grain toast spread with 1 tsp. trans free margarine or light butter (such as Land O'Lakes Light Butter with Canola Oil), sprinkled with ¼ tsp. cinnamon.

Calories: 410
Protein: 17 g
Carbohydrate: 73 g
Fiber: 9 g
Total Fat: 8 g

Saturated Fat: 3 g
Cholesterol: 15 mg
Calcium: 505 mg
Sodium: 330 mg

Lower-Carb Option: Skip the toast and have 1 part-skim cheese stick.

BANANAS FOSTER WAFFLES

Toast 2 whole grain waffles. Toss together ⅓ cup sliced banana, 2 tsp. chopped pecans, and 1 tbsp. maple syrup. Spoon over waffles and serve with 1 cup nonfat milk.

Calories: 410
Protein: 17 g
Carbohydrate: 76 g
Fiber: 9 g
Total Fat: 10 g

Saturated Fat: 1 g
Cholesterol: 5 mg
Calcium: 390 mg
Sodium: 410 mg

Lower-Carb Option: Skip this meal.

WAFFLES WITH PEACHES AND HONEY

Toast 2 whole grain waffles. In a nonstick skillet, sauté 1 sliced peach in 1 tsp. light butter until just tender, about 3 minutes. Spoon over waffles and top with 1 tbsp. honey mixed with ¼ tsp. allspice. Serve with 1 cup light vanilla soy milk (such as Silk Light).

Calories: 400
Protein: 17 g
Carbohydrate: 76 g
Fiber: 9 g
Total Fat: 7 g

Saturated Fat: 3 g
Cholesterol: 4 mg
Calcium: 375 mg
Sodium: 450 mg

Lower-Carb Option: Skip this meal.

VEGETABLE OMELET

Sauté ¼ cup each sliced mushrooms and chopped red peppers with ½ cup chopped asparagus in a nonstick skillet coated with cooking spray until tender, about 4 minutes. Remove vegetables from skillet and keep warm. In the same skillet, add 1 lightly beaten whole egg and 2 egg whites and cook until just firm (do not scramble). Spoon vegetables on top of egg and sprinkle with 2 tbsp. reduced fat shredded cheddar cheese (such as Cabot 50% Reduced Fat). Fold egg in half and cook until cheese is melted, 1-2 minutes. Serve with 3 oz. lean turkey or chicken sausage, lean ham, or veggie sausage (such as Morningstar Farms Veggie Sausage Patties) and a small piece of fruit such as a plum or tangerine.

Calories: 420
Protein: 40 g
Carbohydrate: 39 g
Fiber: 12 g
Total Fat: 13 g

Saturated Fat: 3 g
Cholesterol: 217 mg
Calcium: 185 mg
Sodium: 700 mg

Lower-Carb Option: Have as is.

BERRY BANANA SMOOTHIE

Combine 1 cup lowfat vanilla yogurt, 1 sliced ripe banana, ½ cup frozen mixed berries, 2 tbsp. wheat germ, and ¼ cup ice cubes in a blender. Blend until smooth. Serve with 1 slice whole grain toast spread with 1½ tsp. trans free margarine or light butter (such as Land O'Lakes Light Butter with Canola Oil).

Calories: 400
Protein: 20 g
Carbohydrate: 63 g
Fiber: 8 g
Total Fat: 11 g

Saturated Fat: 4 g
Cholesterol: 15 mg
Calcium: 490 mg
Sodium: 340 mg

Lower-Carb Option: Skip the toast and have 3 oz. lean turkey or chicken sausage, lean meat (such as Hormel Natural Choice), or veggie sausage (such as Morningstar Farms Veggie Sausage Patties).

BREAKFAST BURRITO

Sauté ⅓ cup chopped red peppers and ¼ cup chopped onion in a nonstick skillet coated with cooking spray until tender, about 2-3 minutes. Add 1 beaten whole egg and 1 egg white and scramble until cooked through. Spoon into a whole wheat tortilla (around 120 calories), and top with 2 tbsp. shredded reduced fat Colby Jack or cheddar cheese, 1 tbsp. salsa, and roll up. Serve with ½ cup cubed mango mixed with ½ cup lowfat yogurt.

Calories: 410
Protein: 30 g
Carbohydrate: 55 g
Fiber: 9 g
Total Fat: 9 g

Saturated Fat: 4 g
Cholesterol: 224 mg
Calcium: 420 mg
Sodium: 600 mg

Lower-Carb Option: Have as is.

EGG SANDWICH

Fry 1 egg in a nonstick skillet coated with cooking spray. Serve on a toasted whole grain English muffin stuffed with 1 slice prosciutto or lean ham and ¼ of a sliced avocado. Serve with a 12 oz. skim latte and 1 cup cubed melon.

Calories: 420
Protein: 26 g
Carbohydrate: 45 g
Fiber: 7 g
Total Fat: 15 g

Saturated Fat: 3 g
Cholesterol: 221 mg
Calcium: 560 mg
Sodium: 620 mg

Lower-Carb Option: Have as is.

BAGEL AND SMOKED SALMON

Spread a 3-inch diameter whole wheat bagel (such as Pepperidge Farm Mini) with 1 tbsp. light vegetable cream cheese. Top with a 1-oz. slice of smoked salmon, 2 thin slices red onion and 1 slice tomato. Serve with ½ cup plain lowfat yogurt (such as Fage Total 0% or Oikos Greek) mixed with 1 tbsp. honey and ⅓ cup mixed dried fruit.

Calories: 400
Protein: 18 g
Carbohydrate: 73 g
Fiber: 7 g
Total Fat: 6 g

Saturated Fat: 3 g
Cholesterol: 22 mg
Calcium: 365 mg
Sodium: 500 mg

Lower-Carb Option: Skip this meal.

STARBUCKS BREAKFAST

Mix together ½ cup dried fruit with 2 tbsp. of roasted almonds. Pair with a Grande (16 oz.) skim latte.

Calories: 390
Protein: 13 g
Carbohydrate: 55 g
Fiber: 8 g
Total Fat: 14 g

Saturated Fat: 3 g
Cholesterol: 17 mg
Calcium: 330 mg
Sodium: 120 mg

Lower-Carb Option: Skip this meal.

450-Calorie Lunches

Create Your Own Lunch: While any recipe or combo of foods that provides around 450 calories will do the trick, to create a balanced 450-calorie lunch simply Pick your Protein (1 portion for carb-lovers, 2 portions for protein-lovers), Pile on Produce (3 portions), Grab Your Grain (2 portions for carb lovers, 1 portion for protein-lovers), and Finish with Fat (1 portion). (See portion info on page 216.)

SMOKED SALMON SALAD

Combine 3 cups mixed greens with ¼ cup thinly sliced red onion, ½ cup grape tomatoes, 1 chopped yellow or red pepper, and ½ cup sliced cucumber. Toss with 2 tsp. olive oil mixed with 1 tbsp. balsamic vinegar and ⅛ tsp. freshly ground black pepper. Top with 3 oz. (about 2-3 slices) smoked salmon and 1 tbsp. crumbled goat cheese. Serve with 1 cup berries and 1 tbsp. almonds.

Calories: 460
Protein: 27 g
Carbohydrate: 44 g
Fiber: 11 g
Total Fat: 22 g

Saturated Fat: 5 g
Cholesterol: 26 mg
Calcium: 209 mg
Sodium: 750 mg

Lower-Carb Option: Have as is.

CHICKPEA AND CHICKEN SALAD

Combine 1 cup roasted and chopped skinless, boneless chicken breast (such as Hormel Natural Choice Carved Chicken Breast), ½ cup drained and rinsed low sodium chickpeas (such as Goya Low Sodium), ½ cup halved grape tomatoes, 2 tbsp. chopped fresh basil, and 2 tbsp. shredded Parmesan cheese. Whisk together 2 tbsp. white wine vinegar with 1 tsp. olive oil, 1 tsp. Dijon mustard, 1 clove chopped garlic and ⅛ tsp. black pepper. Drizzle dressing over chicken mixture and 2 cups mixed greens and toss to combine.

Calories: 460
Protein: 56 g
Carbohydrate: 30 g
Fiber: 11 g
Total Fat: 13 g

Saturated Fat: 4 g
Cholesterol: 126 mg
Calcium: 270 mg
Sodium: 430 mg

Lower-Carb Option: Have as is.

COBB SALAD

Combine ½ cup roasted and chopped skinless, boneless chicken breast (such as Hormel Natural Choice Carved Chicken Breast) with 3 cups baby spinach, 1 tbsp. crumbled goat cheese, 1 piece of crumbled bacon, ¼ of an avocado diced, ¼ cup chopped red onion, and ¼ cup cooked corn kernels. Whisk together 2 tbsp. white wine vinegar with 1 tsp. olive oil, 1 tsp. Dijon mustard, 1 clove chopped garlic and ⅛ tsp. black pepper and drizzle over salad. Serve with a small piece of fruit such as a plum or tangerine.

Calories: 450
Protein: 30 g
Carbohydrate: 37 g
Fiber: 9 g
Total Fat: 22 g

Saturated Fat: 5 g
Cholesterol: 67 mg
Calcium: 187 mg
Sodium: 320 mg

Lower-Carb Option: Have as is.

TUNA ENGLISH MUFFINS

Combine 3 oz. albacore tuna packed in water (drained) with 2 tbsp. dried cranberries, 1 tbsp. chopped walnuts, ¼ cup chopped celery, 2 tsp. light mayonnaise (such as Hellmann's Light) and 1 tsp. Dijon mustard. Serve open-faced on a toasted light whole grain English muffin (such as Thomas' Light Multigrain) topped with 2 leafy green lettuce leaves. Serve with 2 cups mixed greens, ½ cup grape or cherry tomatoes, and ½ cup sliced cucumbers with 10-15 sprays spray-able vinaigrette (such as Wishbone Salad Spritzers).

Calories: 440
Protein: 28 g
Carbohydrate: 50 g
Fiber: 12 g
Total Fat: 19 g

Saturated Fat: 2 g
Cholesterol: 36 mg
Calcium: 186 mg
Sodium: 620 mg

Lower-Carb Option: Have as is.

CHICKEN BLT

Spread 1 tsp. light mayonnaise (such as Hellmann's Light) on one slice of toasted whole grain bread. Top with 3 oz. roasted and sliced skinless, boneless chicken breast (such as Hormel Natural Choice Carved Chicken Breast), 1 slice bacon, 2 slices tomato, and 1 cup mixed greens. Top with another slice toasted whole grain bread. Serve with ½ cup lowfat yogurt and ½ cup cubed melon.

Calories: 450
Protein: 42 g
Carbohydrate: 45 g
Fiber: 7 g
Total Fat: 11 g

Saturated Fat: 4 g
Cholesterol: 88 mg
Calcium: 323 mg
Sodium: 610 mg

Lower-Carb Option: Have as is.

HUMMUS AND VEGETABLES

Stuff a small (4 to 5-inch) whole wheat pita (around 80 calories) with
⅓ cup hummus, ½ cup shredded carrots, 1 cup red pepper slices, 1 cup
cucumber slices, and ⅓ an avocado. Serve with an orange.

Calories: 440
Protein: 12 g
Carbohydrate: 68 g
Fiber: 15 g
Total Fat: 15 g

Saturated Fat: 2 g
Cholesterol: 0 mg
Calcium: 142 mg
Sodium: 350 mg

Lower-Carb Option: Skip the pita and dip the vegetables in ½ cup of
hummus.

WALDORF SALAD

Combine 1½ cup broccoli slaw (such as Mann's), 1 cup roasted and
chopped skinless, boneless chicken breast (such as Hormel Natural Choice
Carved Chicken Breast), 1 cup chopped Granny Smith apple (about 1
small), ¼ cup halved seedless grapes, 1 tbsp. chopped walnuts, and 1 tbsp.
bleu cheese. Combine 3 tbsp. plain lowfat yogurt (such as Fage Total 0%
or Oikos Greek), mixed with 1 tbsp. lemon juice, and ⅛ tsp. black pepper.
Serve over 2 cups mixed greens.

Calories: 460
Protein: 51 g
Carbohydrate: 32 g
Fiber: 9 g
Total Fat: 16 g

Saturated Fat: 4 g
Cholesterol: 120 mg
Calcium: 315 mg
Sodium: 420 mg

Lower-Carb Option: Have as is.

AVOCADO VEGETABLE WRAP

Spread a whole wheat tortilla (around 120 calories) with 1 tbsp. reduced fat vegetable cream cheese. Top with 1 cup fresh spinach, ⅓ cup chopped tomatoes, ¼ cup shredded carrots, ¼ sliced avocado, and 1 tbsp. chopped Kalamata olives. Drizzle with 1 tbsp. balsamic vinegar and 2 tsp. chopped fresh basil, and roll up. Serve with ½ cup berries and 1 tbsp. almonds.

Calories: 440
Protein: 14 g
Carbohydrate: 53 g
Fiber: 14 g
Total Fat: 21 g

Saturated Fat: 3 g
Cholesterol: 8 mg
Calcium: 160 mg
Sodium: 500 mg

Lower-Carb Option: Have as is.

VEGETABLE QUESADILLA

In a nonstick skillet, sauté ¼ cup chopped onion and 3 minced garlic cloves in 1 tsp. olive oil until just tender, about 3 minutes. Stir in ½ cup chopped broccoli florets and ½ cup sliced mushrooms and cook until tender, about 5 minutes. Remove vegetables from pan. Coat the same skillet with cooking spray and lay a whole wheat tortilla (around 120 calories) in the skillet. Spoon vegetable mixture onto one half of the tortilla, and top with ⅓ cup shredded reduced fat cheddar cheese (such as Cabot 50% Reduced Fat). Fold the tortilla over the vegetables, and cook until browned, about 4 minutes per side. Top with 2 tbsp. reduced fat sour cream and 2 tbsp. salsa. Serve 3 cups mixed greens tossed with ½ cup grape tomatoes, ½ cup sliced red pepper, and ½ cup sliced cucumber with 10-15 sprays spray-able vinaigrette (such as Wishbone Salad Spritzers) and a small piece of fruit such as a plum or tangerine.

Calories: 450
Protein: 24 g
Carbohydrate: 66 g
Fiber: 15 g
Total Fat: 13 g

Saturated Fat: 4 g
Cholesterol: 23 mg
Calcium: 415 mg
Sodium: 720 mg

Lower-Carb Option: Skip this meal.

ROASTED BEET SALAD

Combine 3 cups mixed greens with 1 chopped pear, 1 tbsp. bleu cheese, 1 tbsp. chopped walnuts, and 1 cup chopped cooked beets (such as Melissa's Baby Beets, or roast your own at 425° for about 45 minutes). Mix together 1 tbsp. orange juice with 1 tbsp. white wine vinegar, 1 tbsp. chopped shallots, 2 tsp. canola oil and ⅛ tsp. black pepper and toss with the salad. Serve with a whole wheat dinner roll (around 100 calories) and a small piece of fruit such as a plum or tangerine.

Calories: 440
Protein: 11 g
Carbohydrate: 67 g
Fiber: 13 g
Total Fat: 17 g

Saturated Fat: 5 g
Cholesterol: 25 mg
Calcium: 323 mg
Sodium: 510 mg

Lower-Carb Option: Skip the roll and have 3 oz. cooked lean meat, fish, shellfish, skinless poultry or 6 oz. tofu.

CARIBBEAN CHICKEN WRAP

Combine 3 oz. roasted and chopped skinless, boneless chicken breast (such as Hormel Natural Choice Carved Chicken Breast) with 2 tbsp. chopped red onion, 2 chopped garlic cloves, ½ cup cubed mango, ¼ cup drained and rinsed low sodium black beans (such as Goya Low Sodium), a pinch of red pepper flakes, and 2 tsp. chopped cilantro. Spoon into a whole wheat tortilla (around 120 calories) and roll up. Serve with 2 tbsp. roasted macadamia nuts and 2 cups of mixed greens with 10-15 sprays spray-able vinaigrette (such as Wishbone Salad Spritzers).

Calories: 450
Protein: 25 g
Carbohydrate: 58 g
Fiber: 15 g
Total Fat: 15 g

Saturated Fat: 2 g
Cholesterol: 35 mg
Calcium: 138 mg
Sodium: 600 mg

Lower-Carb Option: Skip the tortilla, have another 3 oz. chicken, and serve the chicken salad on the mixed greens.

MEDITERRANEAN COUSCOUS

Combine ¾ cup cooked whole wheat couscous with ½ cup rinsed and drained low sodium canellini beans (such as Goya Low Sodium), ¼ cup chopped red onion, ½ cup halved grape tomatoes, and ¼ cup canned, marinated artichoke hearts. Drizzle with 3 tbsp. lemon juice, 1 tsp. olive oil, 2 tbsp. chopped fresh basil and 2 tbsp. crumbled feta cheese. Season with freshly ground pepper and a sprinkle of sea salt. Serve with a small piece of fruit such as a plum or tangerine.

Calories: 440   Saturated Fat: 4 g
Protein: 19 g   Cholesterol: 16 mg
Carbohydrate: 77 g   Calcium: 227 mg
Fiber: 19 g   Sodium: 460 mg
Total Fat: 13 g

Lower-Carb Option: Have just ⅓ cup couscous and have 3 oz. cooked lean meat, fish, shellfish, skinless poultry or 6 oz. tofu.

QUICK TORTELLINI

Sauté 2 chopped garlic cloves, 1 cup sliced portobello mushrooms, ¾ cup halved cherry tomatoes, and ½ cup (frozen, thawed) peas in a non-stick skillet coated with cooking spray until mushrooms are tender, about 5 minutes. Add 2 cups fresh spinach and sauté until wilted, about 1-2 minutes. Toss with 1 cup cooked fresh cheese tortellini (such as Buitoni 3-Cheese) and top with 3 tbsp. grated Parmesan cheese and 1 tbsp. pine nuts. Season with freshly ground pepper and a sprinkle of sea salt. Serve with 2 cups mixed greens with 10-15 sprays spray-able vinaigrette (such as Wishbone Salad Spritzers).

Calories: 460   Saturated Fat: 5 g
Protein: 28 g   Cholesterol: 47 mg
Carbohydrate: 56 g   Calcium: 383 mg
Fiber: 13 g   Sodium: 600 mg
Total Fat: 17 g

Lower-Carb Option: Have just ⅓ cup tortellini and have 3 oz. cooked lean meat, fish, shellfish, skinless poultry or 6 oz. tofu.

FROZEN MEAL LUNCH

Cook one whole grain frozen entrée of your choice (with around 250 calories and at least 3 grams of fiber—such as Lean Cuisine Spa Cuisine). Serve with 1 cup cubed melon and a salad with 3 cups baby lettuce, ½ cup sugar snap peas, ½ cup shredded carrots mixed with 2 tsp. sesame oil, and a splash of white wine vinegar.

Calories: 450
Protein: 24 g
Carbohydrate: 60 g
Fiber: 13 g
Total Fat: 14 g

Saturated Fat: 2 g
Cholesterol: 40 mg
Calcium: 214 mg
Sodium: 650 mg

Lower-Carb Option: Skip this meal.

SUSHI LUNCH

Combine 8 pieces fish and vegetable sushi roll (such as salmon or tuna and cucumber, or California roll) with 1 cup cooked edamame (in pod—½ cup shelled). Serve with an orange.

Calories: 470
Protein: 25 g
Carbohydrate: 83 g
Fiber: 9 g
Total Fat: 5 g

Saturated Fat: 1 g
Cholesterol: 15 mg
Calcium: 135 mg
Sodium: 450 mg

Lower-Carb Option: Have just 4 pieces of the sushi roll and have 5 pieces sashimi.

550-Calorie Dinners

Create Your Own Dinner: While any recipe or combo of foods that provides around 550 calories will do the trick, to create a balanced 550-calorie dinner simply Pick your Protein (1 portion for carb-lovers, 2 portions for protein-lovers), Pile on Produce (3 portions), Grab Your Grain (2 portions for carb lovers, 1 portion for protein-lovers), and Finish with Fat (2 portions). (See portion info on page 216.)

SAUCY CHICKEN WITH PASTA

Sauté ¼ cup chopped onion with 3 chopped garlic cloves in a nonstick skillet coated with cooking spray until soft, about 3 minutes. Add 1 chopped skinless, boneless chicken thighs, ½ cup canned, chopped tomatoes with basil (such as Muir Glen), and ½ tsp. black pepper. Cover and simmer 10 minutes or until chicken is cooked through. Spoon over 1 cup cooked whole wheat or whole grain pasta (such as Barilla Whole Grain) and top with 1 tbsp. grated Parmesan cheese and 1 tbsp. chopped fresh basil. Season with freshly ground pepper and a sprinkle of sea salt. Serve with 2 cups mixed greens, ½ cup grape tomatoes and 1 tbsp. pines nuts with 10-15 sprays spray-able vinaigrette (such as Wishbone Salad Spritzers).

Calories: 560
Protein: 35 g
Carbohydrate: 67 g
Fiber: 10 g
Total Fat: 18 g

Saturated Fat: 3 g
Cholesterol: 63 mg
Calcium: 191 mg
Sodium: 730 mg

Lower-Carb Option: Have just ½ cup of pasta and have another chicken thigh.

BROILED FISH WITH MANGO SALSA

Season 6 oz. orange roughy fillet (or other firm white fish such as halibut or bass) with ⅛ tsp. each garlic powder, salt, black pepper, and cumin. Broil or grill 10 minutes or until fish flakes easily with a fork. Combine ½ cup diced mango with 2 tbsp. chopped red onion, 1 tbsp. chopped red pepper, 1 chopped garlic clove, 2 tsp. chopped cilantro, 2 tbsp. lime juice, and ⅛ tsp. hot sauce. Spoon over fish and serve on top of 1 cup cooked brown rice (such as Uncle Ben's Ready Rice) and ½ cup each sliced zucchini and summer squash sautéed in 2 tsp. olive oil.

Calories: 560
Protein: 47 g
Carbohydrate: 66 g
Fiber: 8 g
Total Fat: 13 g

Saturated Fat: 2 g
Cholesterol: 136 mg
Calcium: 88 mg
Sodium: 450 mg

Lower-Carb Option: Have just ½ cup cooked brown rice and have another 2 ounces of fish.

SPICED SALMON FILLET

Rub a 6 oz. salmon fillet with 2 tsp. brown sugar, 1 tsp. Dijon mustard, ½ tsp. each cumin, coriander, and garlic powder, and ⅛ tsp. salt. Drizzle with 2 tsp. lemon juice and grill or broil 10-15 minutes or until fish flakes easily with a fork. Top with 2 tbsp. chopped green onions. Serve over 1 cup whole wheat couscous and with 1½ cups steamed sugar snap peas, and for dessert ½ cup of raspberries.

Calories: 550
Protein: 44 g
Carbohydrate: 66 g
Fiber: 12 g
Total Fat: 12 g

Saturated Fat: 2 g
Cholesterol: 94 mg
Calcium: 118 mg
Sodium: 500 mg

Lower-Carb Option: Have just ½ cup couscous and have another 2 oz. of salmon.

SHRIMP WITH YOGURT SAUCE

In a medium skillet coated with cooking spray, sauté 5 oz. peeled and deveined shrimp and 1 tbsp. chopped shallots in 1 tbsp. olive oil until cooked through and opaque, about 3-4 minutes. In a small bowl, combine ¼ cup plain lowfat yogurt (such as Fage Total 0%) with 1 tbsp. lemon juice, 1 tsp. honey, 1 tsp. curry powder, ¼ tsp. each cumin, coriander, and cayenne pepper, and ⅛ tsp. salt. Drizzle yogurt sauce over shrimp and toss with 1½ cups steamed cauliflower and top with 2 tbsp. chopped green onions. Season with freshly ground pepper and a sprinkle of sea salt. Serve over 1 cup cooked whole wheat couscous.

Calories: 550
Protein: 43 g
Carbohydrate: 65 g
Fiber: 14 g
Total Fat: 12 g

Saturated Fat: 2 g
Cholesterol: 93 mg
Calcium: 118 mg
Sodium: 500 mg

Lower-Carb Option: Have just ½ cup couscous and have 2 tbsp. peanuts.

SKILLET JAMBALAYA

In a large non-stick skillet coated with cooking spray, sauté ½ cup each diced green pepper and onion, and 1 chopped celery stalk in 1 tsp. olive oil until just tender, about 3 minutes. Add 1 chopped garlic clove, 1 cup sliced zucchini, and 1 small chopped red pepper and sauté 3-4 minutes. Stir in 2 oz. diced, cooked turkey sausage, ½ cup canned diced tomatoes (such as Muir Glen), ¼ tsp. Cajun seasoning (such as McCormick), and ⅛ tsp. cayenne pepper and simmer 5 minutes. Add 1 cup cooked brown rice and cook for 1 minute or until heated through. Serve with 2 cups mixed greens tossed with 2 tsp. olive oil a splash of white wine vinegar.

Calories: 542
Protein: 21 g
Carbohydrate: 78 g
Fiber: 12 g
Total Fat: 18 g

Saturated Fat: 3 g
Cholesterol: 33 mg
Calcium: 162 mg
Sodium: 860 mg

Lower-Carb Option: Have just ½ cup rice and have another 2 oz. turkey sausage.

ROSEMARY PORK WITH APPLES

Season 4 oz. pork tenderloin with ½ tsp. rosemary garlic seasoning (such as Spice Island Adjustable Grinders). Broil for 10-12 minutes or until cooked through. Sauté 1 sliced Granny Smith apple in ½ tbsp. light butter for 2 minutes. Stir in ¼ tsp. cinnamon and 2 tsp. honey, and cook 1 minute. Toss 3 cups broccoli slaw (such as Mann's) with 1 sliced red pepper, 1 chopped garlic clove, 3 tbsp. cider vinegar, 2 tsp. canola oil, and ⅛ tsp. each salt and black pepper. Serve with ½ cup steamed green beans.

Calories: 540
Protein: 41 g
Carbohydrate: 56 g
Fiber: 15 g
Total Fat: 19 g

Saturated Fat: 5 g
Cholesterol: 96 mg
Calcium: 190 mg
Sodium: 610 mg

Lower-Carb Option: Have as is.

HERBED CHICKEN SALAD

Slice a 6 oz. skinless, boneless chicken breast into strips. Toss with 1 tsp. olive oil, 1 tsp. chopped fresh rosemary (or ¼ tsp. dried) and 1 chopped garlic clove. Broil or grill until cooked through, about 8-10 minutes. Combine 3 cups mixed greens with ½ cup chopped tomatoes, ½ cup sliced cucumber, ½ a Granny Smith apple, chopped, and 2 tbsp. slivered almonds. Top with the chicken and 2 tbsp. crumbled goat cheese. Combine 2 tsp. olive oil with 2 tbsp. red wine vinegar, ⅛ tsp. each salt and pepper, and drizzle over salad.

Calories: 560
Protein: 53 g
Carbohydrate: 22 g
Fiber: 8 g
Total Fat: 29 g

Saturated Fat: 7 g
Cholesterol: 120 mg
Calcium: 278 mg
Sodium: 530 mg

Lower-Carb Option: Have as is.

SHRIMP AND ASPARAGUS PASTA

In a medium pan, sauté 6 oz. peeled and deveined shrimp in 2 tsp. olive oil with 2 chopped garlic cloves, and ¼ tsp. fresh ground black pepper until almost cooked through, about 3 minutes. Add ¼ lb. asparagus spears cut into 1-inch pieces (about 1½ cups) cooking until asparagus is tender (about 3 minutes). Stir in 1 tsp. chopped fresh thyme, 1 tbsp. chopped prosciutto, and 2 tbsp. fresh lemon juice. Mix with ½ cup cooked whole wheat or whole grain pasta (such as Barilla Whole Grain) and season with freshly ground pepper and a sprinkle of sea salt. Serve with ½ cup cubed honeydew melon.

Calories: 540
Protein: 49 g
Carbohydrate: 53 g
Fiber: 10 g
Total Fat: 15 g

Saturated Fat: 2 g
Cholesterol: 268 mg
Calcium: 158 mg
Sodium: 650 mg

Lower-Carb Option: Have as is.

BURGER AND FRIES

Season 4 oz. ground turkey with ½ tsp. garlic powder, ½ tsp. onion powder, 1 tsp. Worcestershire sauce and ¼ tsp. black pepper. Form into patty and broil or grill until cooked through, about 7-10 minutes. Serve turkey burger on a toasted whole wheat Kaiser roll (around 200 calories—such as Pepperidge Farms Soft Whole Wheat Kaiser) with 1 tbsp. mustard, 1 slice each tomato, Vidalia onion, and reduced fat Swiss cheese. Serve with 3 oz. baked sweet potato French fries (such as Alexia) and 2 cups mixed greens and ½ cup grape tomatoes topped with 10-15 sprays spray-able vinaigrette (such as Wishbone Salad Spritzers).

Calories: 540
Protein: 42 g
Carbohydrate: 60 g
Fiber: 9 g
Total Fat: 15 g

Saturated Fat: 5 g
Cholesterol: 100 mg
Calcium: 408 mg
Sodium: 800 mg

Lower-Carb Option: Have another 3 oz. ground turkey and serve the burger open-faced on just ½ of the roll.

TOMATO MUSHROOM PASTA

Sauté 1 cup each chopped tomatoes, Portobello mushrooms, and zucchini with 2 chopped garlic cloves, a pinch of salt and ¼ tsp. pepper in a medium skillet coated with cooking spray until tender. Add ½ cup rinsed and drained low sodium canellini beans (such as Goya Low Sodium) and cook until heated through, about 3 minutes. Toss with 1 cup cooked whole wheat or whole grain rotini pasta (such as Barilla Whole Grain) and sprinkle with 1 tablespoons bleu cheese (such as gorgonzola). Season with freshly ground pepper and a sprinkle of sea salt. Serve with 2 cups mixed greens topped with 10-15 sprays spray-able vinaigrette (such as Wishbone Salad Spritzers).

Calories: 560
Protein: 32 g
Carbohydrate: 98 g
Fiber: 22 g
Total Fat: 8 g

Saturated Fat: 3 g
Cholesterol: 11 mg
Calcium: 313 mg
Sodium: 670 mg

Lower-Carb Option: Have just ½ cup pasta and have another ¼ cup beans.

MEDITERRANEAN CHICKEN

In a medium skillet coated with cooking spray, cook 2 chopped skinless, boneless chicken thighs until cooked through, about 10 minutes. Add ½ cup canned, drained and chopped artichoke hearts, ¼ cup chopped tomatoes, 1 tbsp. chopped Kalamata olives, and cook until warmed through. Top with 1 tbsp. feta cheese and 2 tbsp. chopped basil. Serve over ¾ cup cooked whole wheat couscous and season with freshly ground pepper and a sprinkle of sea salt. Serve with 1 cup arugula mixed with ¼ an avocado and 1 tbsp. thinly sliced red onion topped with 5-10 sprays spray-able vinaigrette (such as Wishbone Salad Spritzers).

Calories: 560
Protein: 41 g
Carbohydrate: 48 g
Fiber: 11 g
Total Fat: 25 g

Saturated Fat: 7 g
Cholesterol: 140 mg
Calcium: 266 mg
Sodium: 750 mg

Lower-Carb Option: Have as is.

SCALLOPS WITH PASTA

In a medium skillet, sear 5 oz. scallops seasoned with ⅛ tsp. each salt and pepper in 1 tbsp. olive oil until just browned. Add ¼ cup dry white wine, 3 cloves chopped garlic, 1 tsp. capers (or chopped green olives). Cook 3 minutes or until scallops are cooked through. Toss with 1 cup whole wheat or whole grain fettuccini (such as Barilla Whole Grain), 1 tbsp. fresh thyme and 1 cup summer squash sautéed in a nonstick skillet coated with cooking spray. Season with freshly ground pepper and a sprinkle of sea salt. Serve with 2 cups mixed greens topped with 10-15 sprays spray-able vinaigrette (such as Wishbone Salad Spritzers).

Calories: 550
Protein: 35 g
Carbohydrate: 57 g
Fiber: 10 g
Total Fat: 18 g

Saturated Fat: 2 g
Cholesterol: 47 mg
Calcium: 126 mg
Sodium: 730 mg

Lower-Carb Option: Have just ½ cup pasta and have another 3 oz. scallops.

SEARED ASIAN TUNA

Sprinkle a 4 oz. tuna steak with ½ tsp. black pepper and 1 tbsp. sesame seeds. In a nonstick pan coated with cooking spray, sear the tuna for 2-3 minutes on each side. Remove from pan. Sauté 1 cup broccoli, 1 cup sugar snap peas, and ½ cup slices red pepper in 2 tsp. sesame oil until just tender. Toss with 1 tbsp. lite soy sauce and ¼ tsp. red pepper flakes. Serve with ¾ cup cooked brown rice (such as Uncle Ben's Ready Rice).

Calories: 550
Protein: 38 g
Carbohydrate: 48 g
Fiber: 9 g
Total Fat: 23 g

Saturated Fat: 3 g
Cholesterol: 45 mg
Calcium: 150 mg
Sodium: 700 mg

Lower-Carb Option: Have as is.

SIMPLE ROASTED CHICKEN

Coat a 4 oz. skinless, boneless chicken breast in 1 chopped garlic clove and ¼ tsp. rosemary garlic seasoning (such as Spice Island Adjustable Grinders). Roast at 400° for 15 to 20 minutes or until chicken is cooked through. Serve with 1 cup broccoli and 1 cup sugar snap peas sautéed in 1 tbsp. olive oil, 1 whole wheat dinner roll (around 100 calories), and an apple.

Calories: 540
Protein: 43 g
Carbohydrate: 49 g
Fiber: 10 g
Total Fat: 20 g

Saturated Fat: 3 g
Cholesterol: 96 mg
Calcium: 139 mg
Sodium: 360 mg

Lower-Carb Option: Have as is.

SIMPLE ROASTED SALMON

Rub a 5 oz. salmon fillet with 1 chopped garlic clove and ⅛ tsp. each salt and pepper. Drizzle with 1 tbsp. lemon juice and roast at 400° for 15 minutes or until salmon is cooked through. Serve with 2 cups baby spinach sautéed in 1 tsp. olive oil and topped with 1 tbsp. pine nuts, 1 whole wheat dinner roll (around 100 calories), and a peach.

Calories: 540
Protein: 36 g
Carbohydrate: 30 g
Fiber: 6
Total Fat: 31 g

Saturated Fat: 5 g
Cholesterol: 84 mg
Calcium: 122 mg
Sodium: 270 mg

Lower-Carb Option: Have as is.

150-Calorie Snacks

Create Your Own Snack: While any snack (fruit, veggies, nuts, a fiber-rich bar, whole grain crackers, whole grain cereal, etc.) that provides around 150 calories will do the trick, a calcium-rich pick is your best bet. Until 50 years of age women need a daily dose of 1,000 mg of calcium, and from 51 on, 1,200 mg. This bone-building mineral is essential for good health and unfortunately most women come up short in reaching their daily needs. The 150-calorie snacks below provide between 200 to 300 mg of calcium. This, along with the calcium in your meals should get you close to your daily calcium needs, however, to play it safe I suggest you take a multi (see page 219) that provides around 200 mg of calcium (if you are 51 or over you'll need to take a calcium supplement with 200 – 500 mg of calcium in addition to your multi.)

- 1 sliced pear with 1 oz. reduced fat cheese
- 1 sliced apple with 1 oz. reduced fat cheese
- 1 cup of light chocolate soymilk with 1 cup of raspberries
- 1 cup of light vanilla soymilk with 1 sliced peach
- ½ cup lowfat yogurt topped with 1 tbsp. chopped pistachios and 1 tsp. honey
- 1 sliced apple dipped in ½ cup nonfat ricotta sprinkled with cinnamon
- 1 cup of whole strawberries dipped in ½ cup nonfat ricotta drizzled with 1 tsp. honey
- ½ cup lowfat yogurt mixed with 1 tbsp. dried fruit and 1 tbsp slivered almonds
- ½ cup lowfat yogurt with fruit (1 cup of berries or 1 medium sized fruit like an apple, an orange or banana)

- Starbucks Grande Skinny Latte (any flavor) (or any 16 oz. latte with nonfat milk)
- 4 reduced fat Triscuits crackers with and 1 oz. reduced fat cheese
- Fruity Smoothie: blend ¾ cup calcium-fortified orange juice, ½ cup strawberries, ½ small banana, and ¼ cup ice until combined
- Creamy Smoothie: blend ¾ cup vanilla soy milk, ½ cup each blueberries and raspberries until combined
- Veggie Dip: ½ cup plain lowfat yogurt mixed with 1 tsp. lemon juice and ¼ tsp. fresh mint served with 1½ cups sliced veggies, such as carrots, red pepper, and cucumber
- 1 oz. reduced fat cheese and 1 cup grapes
- 1 cup fat free milk and 4 small graham cracker squares

100-Calorie Craving Tamers

Feel like snacking on chips? Go for it. Craving chocolate? Dig in. Dreaming of ice cream? Help yourself. Craving Tamers help you keep your food cravings in check by simply slimming down the portions. A 100-calorie Craving Tamer of anything you want will give you the taste you crave, but without the damage. If you want to save up your Craving Tamer calories and have around 200 calories every other day, or have all 700 calories one day of the week, that's fine too. Or, if you want to cut calories a bit more and skip them altogether, that works as well.

- Skinny Cow Skinny Dipper or Fat Free Fudge Bar
- A 100-calorie pack of anything
- Edy's Frozen Fruit Bar
- 1 sliced apple dipped in a tbsp. of caramel or butterscotch
- 1 cup of berries topped with 4 tbsp. of fat free Reddi-Wip
- 3 ginger snaps
- ½ cup of sorbet
- ½ cup of low fat ice cream or frozen yogurt
- 4 Hershey's Kisses
- 4 mini Three Musketeers
- 2 Hershey's Miniatures
- 2 Miniature Reese's Peanut Butter Cups
- 2 oz. VitaMuffin

- 1 fat free pudding cup
- 10 baked tortilla chips with ¼ cup salsa
- 3 handfuls of unbuttered popcorn
- 1 slice Pepperidge Farm Raisin Cinnamon Swirl Bread with 1 tsp light butter
- 1 cup of sliced strawberries topped with 1 tbsp. fat free hot fudge
- 12 oz. light beer or a 5 oz. glass of wine

For more good food finds and extra help navigating the supermarket aisles, check out www.GroceryCartMakeover.com.

Closing Thoughts...

Heather...

I'm not going to pretend that everything you need for the rest of your healthy life can be squeezed into one book. The fact is there are lots of other super helpful resources out there that can help you stay on top of your health game. There are healthy-living magazines and nutrition newsletters (I think the *Nutrition Action Healthletter* is a must-have for anyone concerned about their health), e-newsletters (I love the invaluable product reviews in the fun, free e-newsletter from the www.hungry-girl.com), restaurants helpers (my favs are the books *Restaurant Confidential* by Michael F. Jacobson and Jayne Hurley and *Eat This, Not That* by David Zinczenko and Matt Goulding, grocery store guides (*The Grocery Cart Makeover*, created by yours truly, will help you fill your cart with the best choices—www. grocerycartmakeover.com), exercise books (*Get With the Program* by Bob Greene and *Bob Greene's Total Body Makeover*) and tons of healthy cookbooks and magazines.

However, this book is a sure-fire way to help you understand yourself, and in turn understand the best ways for you to shake those extra pounds and start living a happier and healthier life! Unlike other "diet" books that ask you to change who you are and follow their plan, *What's Your Diet Type* explains how you can work with your own unique strengths and weaknesses to lose weight and feel better for a lifetime.

Ed...

Over the past 18 years of medical practice I have seen diets come, and I've seen diets go. Some of these diets were medically sound (whatever *that* means!) and some not so much. The thing is, all diets work for some of the people some of the time. I've not come across a specific diet that works for all people all of the time. This tells me one thing; either medical science hasn't found the one "secret" diet that works for everyone—or more likely, the secret truly is matching the person with *the diet that will work for them*. Herein lies the magic of this book. You, the reader, have your own particular likes and dislikes and I think (my personal opinion) that the diet industry is somewhat arrogant stating that you must fit your life around their diet. Perhaps a better approach would be to find a diet that fits around your life. You are unique as your fingerprint. How can you make sure your diet is too? Reading and applying the concepts in this book is a great way to start.

I have seen patients with seemingly "incurable" conditions recover fully. I have observed individuals that have been told that they will have to take medicine for the rest of their lives get off their medications and thrive. I have witnessed people that were told that they would never walk again go on to run marathons. I have had the joy of meeting people that have "tried and failed every diet" tap into the strengths of their Diet Type and achieve their weight goals. The human spirit—once ignited—is the strongest force in the universe. I encourage you to light your spirit, ignite your passion, and engage your unstoppable determination. Once you do, the future is yours to shape. I look forward to hearing your success stories as you follow the path that is right for you. As Frank Sinatra once sang, "I did it my way..."

Mary...

This is more than a diet book. It is a delightfully delicious guide for following your personality to the weight you love. Once you consume and digest the information and concepts in this book, you'll have a greater understanding about what makes you tick. It encourages you get to know and express yourself in ways you may have never thought of before. In the days, weeks and months to come, you will more readily notice whether your values, needs and joys are being met or expressed ways that bring you true satisfaction and happiness. The more you recognize and follow the flow of your personality and unique body rhythms (instead of fighting your nature and stuffing your urges) the better you will feel. The better you feel, the more automatically you'll begin to find and implement more resourceful and gratifying ways to replace previous habits. Instead of mindlessly eating or constantly worrying about calories or fat grams, you'll find that your mind and thoughts are more freed up to concentrate on other endeavors and your energy will increase.

As you continue to uncover and discover more about yourself you'll realize that the best way to achieve and maintain a healthy weight that is RIGHT FOR YOU is to enjoy foods that enliven your well-being and provide vitality and enrichment. You will pay more attention to and appreciate opportunities to move your body and feel the difference it makes when activity is a part of your daily life- like breathing- automatic and life sustaining. Imagine yourself at your ideal weight, enjoying life, feeling good, having great energy for the things that you value most. Keep this picture in your mind and act as if it is truly a reality right now. Before you realize it, that mental picture—when aligned with your true nature (not what you think you *should* or *shouldn't* do, be, or look like) comes into focus and form. What is it you will be doing with the extra time you have that used to be spent worrying about your weight? Have fun exploring, learning and trying out new ways of expressing your personality. If you dive in wholeheartedly, I promise it will be a real adventure!

About the Authors

Heather K. Jones, R.D.

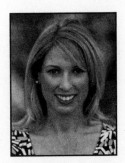

Heather Jones received her Bachelor of Science from the University of Maryland and has been a Registered Dietitian (R.D.) and weight-loss counselor for over ten years. An accomplished freelance journalist, Ms. Jones has been published in many of the nation's leading healthy-living magazines and publications, including *SELF* and *Fitness* Magazine. She is a nutrition consultant for Bob Greene's *The Best Life Diet*, and the author of *The Grocery Cart Makeover*.

Mary Miscisin

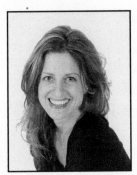

Mary Miscisin received her M.S. in Fitness and Wellness Management and is an expert on psychology and personality with over 20 years of experience facilitating employee wellness programs. She is a certified MBTI® administrator, a True Colors© trainer, and the author of *Showing Our True Colors*, a guide used around the world for understanding and applying the concepts of personality styles.

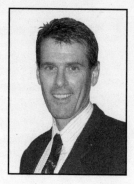

Ed Redard, M.D.

Ed Redard, M.D. received his medical degree from U.C. Davis and has been a Family Practice Physician for over 18 years. As a certified MBTI® administrator and a True Colors© trainer, he is expertly skilled in combining the Personality Theory with modern medicine to guide patients to health and wellness.